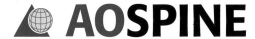

AOSPINE

Jens R Chapman | Michael J Lee | Jeffrey T Hermsmeyer | Joseph R Dettori | Daniel C Norvell

Measurements in Spine Care

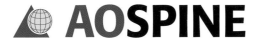

Jens R Chapman | Michael J Lee | Jeffrey T Hermsmeyer | Joseph R Dettori | Daniel C Norvell

Measurements in Spine Care

228 Illustrations

Thieme

Design and layout: nougat GmbH, CH-4056 Basel
Illustrations: nougat GmbH, CH-4056 Basel
Production: AO Publishing, CH-8600 Dübendorf

Library of Congress Cataloging-in-Publication Data is available from the publisher.

Hazards

Great care has been taken to maintain the accuracy of the information contained in this publication. However, the publisher, and/or the distributor, and/or the editors, and/or the authors cannot be held responsible for errors or any consequences arising from the use of the information contained in this publication. Contributions published under the name of individual authors are statements and opinions solely of said authors and not of the publisher, and/or the distributor, and/or the AO Group.

The products, procedures, and therapies described in this work are hazardous and are therefore only to be applied by certified and trained medical professionals in environments specially designed for such procedures. No suggested test or procedure should be carried out unless, in the user's professional judgment, its risk is justified. Whoever applies products, procedures, and therapies shown or described in this work will do this at their own risk. Because of rapid advances in the medical sciences, AO recommends that independent verification of diagnosis, therapies, drugs, dosages, and operation methods should be made before any action is taken.

Although all advertising material which may be inserted into the work is expected to conform to ethical (medical) standards, inclusion in this publication does not constitute a guarantee or endorsement by the publisher regarding quality or value of such product or of the claims made of it by its manufacturer.

Copyright © 2012 by AOSpine International, Switzerland, Stettbachstrasse 6, CH-8600 Dübendorf
Distribution by Georg Thieme Verlag, Rüdigerstrasse 14, DE-70469 Stuttgart and
Thieme New York, 333 Seventh Avenue, New York, NY 10001, USA

ISBN: 9783131711915
E-ISBN: 9783131726513

Contributors

Editors

Jens R Chapman, MD
Department of Orthopedics and
Sports Medicine
Harborview Medical Center
University of Washington
325 Ninth Avenue, ZA-48
Seattle, WA 98104-2499
USA

Michael J Lee, MD
Department of Orthopedics and
Sports Medicine
Harborview Medical Center
University of Washington
1959 NE Pacific Street
Seattle, WA 98195
USA

Jeffrey T Hermsmeyer, BSc
Project Manager
Spectrum Research, Inc.
705 S 9th Street, Suite 203
Tacoma, WA 98405
USA

Joseph R Dettori, PhD, MPH
Spectrum Research, Inc.
705 S 9th Street, Suite 203
Tacoma, WA 98405
USA

Daniel C Norvell, PhD
Spectrum Research, Inc.
705 S 9th Street, Suite 203
Tacoma, WA 98405
USA

Authors

Saumyajit Basu, MS(orth), DNB(orth), FRCSEd
Consultant Spine Surgeon
Park Clinic
4 Gorky Terrace
700017 Kolkata
India

Richard J Bransford, MD
Department of Orthopedics and
Sports Medicine
Harborview Medical Center
University of Washington
325 Ninth Avenue
Seattle, WA 98104-2499
USA

Michael G Fehlings, MD, PhD
Department of Neurosurgery
University of Toronto
4 West, Room 449
399 Bathurst Street
Toronto, Ontario M5T 2S8
Canada

Gregory A Kinney, PhD
Department of Rehabilitation Medicine
University of Washington
325 Ninth Avenue
Seattle, WA 98104-2499
USA

G R Vijay Kumar, MD
Department of Neurosurgery
Institute of Neuroscience Kolkata
185/1, A.J.C. Bose Road
700017 Kolkata
India

Charles Kuntz IV, MD
Department of Neurological Surgery
University of Cincinnati – Mayfield Clinic
1 Camargo Pines Lane
Cincinnati, OH 45243
USA

Paul Licina, MD
Holy Spirit Northside Hospital
627 Rode Road, Chermside
4032 Brisbane
Australia

Quynh T Nguyen, PA-C, MHS
Department of Radiology
Harborview Medical Center
University of Washington
325 Ninth Avenue
Seattle, WA 98104-2499
USA

Jamie Purzner, MD
Department of Neurosurgery
University of Toronto
Toronto Western Hospital
4 West, Room 427
399 Bathurst Street
Toronto, Ontario M5T 2S8
Canada

Teresa Purzner, MD
Department of Neurosurgery
University of Toronto
Toronto Western Hospital
4 West, Room 427
399 Bathurst Street
Toronto, Ontario M5T 2S8
Canada

Gregory J Redding, MD
Pulmonary and Sleep Medicine Division
University of Washington
Seattle Children's Hospital
4800 Sand Point Way NE
Seattle, WA 98105
USA

Christiano E Simões, MD
Department of Orthopedics and
Traumatology
Hospital Felício Rocho
Avenida do Contorno 9530
30110-060 Belo Horizonte
Brazil

Paul Thng, MD
Department of Orthopedic Surgery
Changi General Hospital
2 Simei Street 3
Singapore 529889
Singapore

Gail Van Norman, MD
Department of Anesthesiology and
Pain Medicine
University of Washington
1959 Pacific Street NE
Seattle, WA 98195
USA

Emiliano Vialle, MD
Department of Orthopedics
Catholic University of Parana
Rue Brigadeiro Franco 979
8430210 Curitiba
Brazil

Elizabeth Wako, MD
Department of Anesthesiology and
Pain Medicine
University of Washington
1959 Pacific Street NE
Seattle, WA 98195
USA

Preface

"If every general contractor defined a foot as the length of his own foot, our buildings and the construction industry in general would be in a state of disarray. Yet that is precisely what we have done in health care. Every hospital, practice and specialty society has traditionally measured key processes of health care in unique and differing ways."
– Eugene Beed MD, 1996 HEDIS conference

Measuring, quantifying, and calibrating physical elements and activities through testing are acts of appraisal that hold the promise of improving our understanding of the world around us.

The ability to voluntarily measure or quantify the surrounding world can be described as an innately human achievement. It can be considered a true milestone of evolution when man first started using a reproducible unit-measuring device in order to convey a quantification of an object to his or her fellow man. As civilization has evolved into ever more complex structures, standards of measurements likely have changed from an initial practical option for some humans to an existential necessity for mankind. It is a remarkable feat of human concord that standards of measurement have evolved from a myriad of idiosyncratic coexisting concepts to fewer and more globally accepted systems. This is all the more astounding since at the core of measurement standards lie arbitrarily and nonscientifically selected units, which through the course of time and the power of laws have become the standards by which the world as we know it is being quantified. The meter, for instance, was not based on some scientific findings, but established in Paris, France, by the Conférence générale des poids et mesures (General Conference on Weights and Measures) in the Convention du mètre (Treaty of the Mètre) in 1875.

As we slowly "inch" our way towards the use of more unitarian measurement systems applicable throughout the world, medicine as a principally scientific discipline has been at the forefront of the globalization of unit measures for practicality reasons. Within medicine, the global shift to the metric system has made manifest progress. Imagine if every pharmacist, nurse, and physician had to convert ounces to kilograms, inches to centimeters, and gallons to liters every time an order was issued for a patient. While the conversions are not complex, when done countless times by countless individuals, there is certainly elevated risk for error and unnecessary, preventable harm to patients. As we are witnessing the globalization of medicine in health care and scientific research, it becomes a highly relevant, yet ambitious goal to seek out disease-specific normative data and measurement methods, and then to utilize these same constants across continents and cultures.

The evaluation of spinal disorders has more frequently than not defied attempts at objective measurement. Despite the availability of sophisticated (and very expensive) diagnostic tools that provide unprecedented insights into anatomy and physiology, interpretation of the results remains commonly subjective. Differences in spine-specific clinical measurements can prove to be confusing, particularly as the scientific exchange of ideas becomes increasingly globalized. Unlike measurements of weight, length or volume, which can be converted by a simple multiplier, measurements of spine-specific clinical presentations are often more complex, not only in the measurement technique itself, but also in the clinical utility and scientific validity. For example, consider the assessment of cervical spinal stenosis. This can be assessed through direct measurement from a x-ray, a calculation of a ratio from radiographic measurements, cross-sectional area on MRI, midsagittal diameter as seen on an MRI, or simple qualitative appearance on an MRI. While a cross-sectional area on the MRI may be the most accurate assessment of stenosis, it is also costly, requires computer software for calculation and thus may not be the most useful measure to the clinician.

As our previous book *Spine Classification and Severity Measures* sought to present a compendium and evaluation of currently available spinal classifications, the purpose of this text is to provide a reasonably comprehensive status quo of the prevalent range of spine-specific clinical tests and measurement techniques, which seek to objectively quantify disease states and/or function. We also sought to provide the readership with an objective assessment of the measurement technique itself, using a number of simple criteria. For our evaluation we thought it helpful to look at two distinctly different categories—the entities of scientific validity and clinical utility. Of course, an ideal measurement tool should have both scientific validity and clinical utility. While our methods of describing and evaluating these measurements may not be "validated" in the scientific sense, the paradigm of what we felt constituted an "ideal spine measurement" was developed by a group of experienced spine surgeons, other specialists that work in the area of spine (eg, anesthesiologists), and epidemiologists.

In this text, we present and grade a range of measurement techniques commonly used to assess spine-specific clinical presentation. We have identified scientific and clinical features that are valuable for a spine-specific clinical measure. Clearly, the identification of universal, optimal spine-specificclinical measurements is of great importance not only in patient care, but also for facilitating a common language of communication between clinicians and in designing future clinical studies. One may not necessarily agree with our grades assigned in this text. However, more important is the fact that these measurement tools are being presented in a single source reference, juxtaposed to one another for direct comparison, and critically assessed, which we felt was necessary given the myriad of measurements presented in multiple textbooks and journals. In the end, our hope is that this text may contribute to improved patient care by helping practitioners in spine better understand current available options, raising awareness of options where applicable, and hopefully spurring developments to standardize measurements and to fill in the many gaps we currently have in testing, measuring, and understanding our patients with spinal disorders better.

Michael J Lee
Jens R Chapman

Foreword/Acknowledgments

What really matters

....

"It's not what you look at that matters, it's what you see."
                                        – Henry David Thoreau

The act of measuring something promises resolution to a most basic human endeavor: finding truth. Finding truth in numbers has become an increasingly desirable quality in our times.

At first glance this third book in the AOSpine series *Science in Spine* with the title *Measurements in Spine Care* would seem to be a straightforward undertaking: collect the most well-known metrological tests regarding the spine, which are usually expressed in degrees of angulation, pounds or kilograms, and millimeters or inches. Reality turned out to be quite different. Our second book *Spine Classifications and Severity Measures* revealed the ongoing struggles to categorize spinal ailments. It was a major undertaking but a definable effort. The first book *Spine Outcomes Measures and Instruments* represented a hitherto unprecedented effort at reviewing all spine related outcomes studies—seemingly an impossibly vague task. In the end outcomes tests were arguably the most well-organized and reviewable entities. Most authors of these tests had undertaken credible scientific efforts to formulate and then prove the relevance and validity of their outcomes tests.

In retrospect, the task of systematically assessing outcomes and even the droves of classifications paled in comparison to the identification, categorization, and final evaluation of the myriad of objective clinical measurements obtained through tests. The most basic demand on measurements objectivity turned out to be frequently elusive in even the most basic applications.

Meaningful attempts at quantifying spinal "function" usually remained fuzzy, faddish or frankly nonexistent in any or all domains. Besides some measurements directly relevant to spinal function and health, there exist many "oblique" or indirect tests with quantifications that may reflect limited aspects of "spinal well-being". We found exploring these attempts at measuring and quantifying spinal conditions through objective measurements to be both a fascinating and frustrating undertaking as we migrated through many domains and advances of modern medicine—from simple physical examinations to highly expensive "high-tech" tests. None of the tests we evaluated could claim the distinction of being clearly diagnostic of all or even a majority of spinal conditions in isolation of other modalities. However, we found stark differences in our survey of spine-related measurement approaches regarding health care expenses, discomfort, or outright danger to patients and actual test validity. We conclude with what may sound like a disappointment: we are far from "finding truth" in quantifying and measuring our spines.

As in any book, our authors hope to advance the field of spinal medicine directly with this compendium of spinal measurements and its many different domains. We believe that this book will provide systemic categorizations for what we currently have in our armamentarium to understand the human spine and use the many resources, diagrams, and analyses of this book for the advancement of spine care. We believe that this unprecedented effort by a global multispecialty congregation of AOSpine surgeons will also spur a debate on the next steps: "what really matters" when we look at a patient's spine, so that it may enable us to "see what's wrong".

The editors of this textbook wish to acknowledge the following individuals for their invaluable contributions:

- Our section and chapter authors for their expertise and diligence in reviewing the subject matters at hand and for their faith in and commitment to this project through many years of trials and reviews
- Our core methodologists at Spectrum Inc., Tacoma, Washington, who unfailingly provided support and thoroughness in compiling and then testing the subject matter at hand
- Key members of AOSpine International and also AO Education, led by Urs Rüetschi, who provided inspiration, funding, and most importantly vision and drive for this project. We would also like to recognize in particular Carl Lau for his tireless effort in keeping this project on track, and Sigrid Unterberg for proofreading the book
- The illustration team at Nougat Inc., Basel, in particular Zoe Koh and Rolf Joray for their artistic precision in compiling the most comprehensive and consistent image library related to all things spine, and to Tom Wirth for his invaluable help in the typesetting of this book
- Our families, for their love and understanding for our time spent in pursuit of this project: Shirley, Alexandra, Jed, Lucas, and Eva Chapman; Cathy, Karis and Carson Lee; Luralee Dettori; Shelly, Luke, Sophia, and Kate Norvell; Janel, Evan, and Camryn Hermsmeyer

Jens R Chapman
Michael J Lee
Joseph R Dettori
Daniel C Norvell
Jeffrey T Hermsmeyer

Table of contents

1 Methods for identifying and evaluating quality spine measurements

In our previous two books, *Spine Outcomes Measures and Instruments* and *Spine Classification and Severity Measures*, the measures that we attempted to identify and evaluate were literature driven. We systematically searched the literature for all available measures. Such an approach was beyond the scope of this book since there is an abundance of spine measurements in use today. Therefore, experts in each specialty area were invited to identify all measurements that they felt were common, clinically relevant, and sometimes controversial. Each clinical author was directed to refer to the following three questions when writing their chapter and selecting the measurements to be evaluated:

- What are the most suitable tests or measurements to test disease or trauma with a spine population?
- What are the most reliable screening tests during preoperative evaluation of spine patients?
- What is the scientific basis for the use of these tests and measurements in a spine population?

These measurements were compiled and evaluated for quality in each of the chapters corresponding to the specialty area.

What makes a quality spine measurement?

Many factors must be considered when selecting a "quality spine measurement". An explanation of these factors is the main focus of this chapter. In assessing the overall quality of a spine measurement, two major areas should be considered: scientific validity and clinical utility.

Scientific validity

Our expert panel agreed that a measurement tool should possess the following four methodological qualities:

- Interobserver reliability
- Intraobserver reliability
- Universality
- Disease specificity

The value of interobserver and intraobserver reliability is obvious. If one cannot reliably repeat a measurement, or if a second individual cannot reliably reproduce that measurement, then that measurement has little worth. We have reviewed the literature to assess interobserver and intraobserver reliability for all measurements.

Universality refers to the spectrum of diseases for which a measurement tool can be used. The Adams trunk forward bending test, for instance, could be considered one of the most simple "back tests", being representative of the ability of a patient to lean forward. This test can be performed by any patient with almost any spine condition, and some conclusions as to mobility, flexibility, and trunk conditioning of the patient can be drawn. For certain thoracolumbar scoliotic deformities this test becomes particularly relevant as it will show unilateral trunk elevation indicative of an axial rotational deformity.

Disease specificity reflects the accuracy of the measurement in indicating disease. For example lumbar range of motion is a nonspecific measure, whereas Schober's test may more specifically suggest pathology, such as ankylosing spondylitis or diffuse idiopathic skeletal hyperostosis.

Clinical utility

Our expert panel agreed that a measurement tool ideally should feature these four components of clinical utility:

- Ease of application
- Simplicity
- Patient tolerability
- Affordability

Ease of application refers to the level of difficulty in performing the measurement. Assessing range of motion with a physical exam is clearly easier than utilizing infrared motion sensors.

Simplicity refers to the interpretation of the measurement. If a measurement requires several complex formulaic conversions to yield a meaningful result, then it may not be an ideal measurement.

Patient tolerability is very important in assessing a measurement tool. For example, some patients cannot tolerate an MRI because of claustrophobia. For these patients, supplemental treatments such as anesthesia or alternative measures may need to be utilized. Also, tests that pose actual risks to patients through their invasiveness or induced physiological changes would rank low in the category of patient tolerability. For instance, pneumoencephalography was widely used in the early 20th century to provide brain imaging on plain radiographs, but almost invariably resulted in severe headaches, vomiting, and even death. Fortunately this test has been completely replaced by cranial CT and MRI scans. In contrast to pneumoencephalography, cranial CT and MRI scans would score very high on patient tolerability.

Finally, the role of cost in health care cannot be overstated. Affordability as the measurement of actual cost of a modality compared to the ability of a purchaser to pay for it is an intrinsically fluctuating proposition. We, therefore, used simple categories of price versus benefit for an assumed general target population to estimate the affordability of a number of tests from which measurements for spine related disorders can be derived. The dilemma of affordability in health care can be explained with a lumbar MRI scan, which is a very expensive study. If used for certain diseases it can be very affordable. For instance, for an epidural abscess with lumbar discitis, the diagnostic benefit can be very high. Decisive appropriate care can be initiated without great delay and lasting disability through paralysis and major spinal column destruction can be averted. However, if used for routine low back pain screening, the affordability of MRI would become very low. There would be a very high degree of utilization with unclear therapeutic benefit. In our determination of affordability we could not control for the frequency with which practitioners might utilize a test in question. We used a good faith estimation of the average intended use of any given modality. In the case of lumbar MRI the vast majority of cases reveal no clear surgical pathology and thus the overall affordability of this modality is deemed relatively low. As shown in this example, the affordability category remains an abstract estimation and invites controversy without simple resolution. Yet it is intricately linked to our ability to deliver health care in the future by becoming more cost-conscientious.

2   How the spine measurements are displayed in this book

The purpose of this book is to provide the clinician or researcher with a user-friendly display of many of the most common spine measurements, all in one quick reference text. We chose to provide a short introduction to each of the major spine measurement domains by an expert in the field followed by a summary of each spine measurement relative to that domain.

The spine measurements in this book are divided broadly into three main categories: clinical measurements, laboratory measurements, and radiographic measurements. Each category is further divided into the following subcategories and presented accordingly in the book.

Clinical measurements
- Range of motion
- Neurological
- Strength
- Body composition

Laboratory measurements
- Blood, urine, plasma, and serum
- Electrophysiological
- Pulmonary

Radiographic measurements
- Fractures and dislocations
- Disease
- Deformity

Each subcategory contains an introduction that seeks to explain the development, evolution, and current status of the corresponding spine measurement. These introductions are followed by a summary of the spine measurements found within each subcategory. Where appropriate, we have included illustrations of the spine measurement and a legend, if the illustration needs an explanation.

Each spine measurement is summarized on a double-page spread containing:

- Description of its content, interpretation, and clinical relevance
- Summary of any interobserver or intraobserver reliability evaluations with corresponding patient populations
- Score for scientific component consisting of interobserver and intraobserver reliability, universality, and disease specificity
- Score for clinical utility based on ease of application, simplicity, patient tolerability, and affordability

The content evaluation contains a written description of what makes up the spine measurement. This is followed by how to interpret the measurement. Finally, the clinical relevance of each measurement from the perspective of a spine surgeon is given.

The methodology (interobserver and intraobserver reliability) summary section includes the population in which the spine measurement was tested and whether the measurement was found to be reliable. If there was no such testing found in the literature, then it is listed as "not tested". A "+" symbol indicates that the concept was judged favorably (eg, it was found to have interobserver or intraobserver reliability), while a "–" symbol indicates that it was judged unfavorably (eg, it was found not to have interobserver or intraobserver reliability) in the corresponding population.

The content evaluation, methodology, clinical utility, and overall score sections are also summarized by a "bubble score" depicting the number of points it received out of the total points possible.

3   Clinical measurements
3.1 Range of motion

3   Clinical measurements

3.1   Range of motion

Introduction

Medical measurements are becoming increasingly important with escalating demand from health care payers and consumers for improved clinical outcomes at lower costs. Among the more commonly measured functional parameters are muscle power, endurance, movement patterns, and range of motion of joints [1].

Utility of clinical range of motion measurement
Alteration in the clinical range of motion has historically enabled clinicians to diagnose a disease process and to monitor the progress of treatment. More recently range of motion measurements have been used as a marker for clinical outcome studies, utilization reviews, and for a number of impairment guides in many countries.

What is a good measurement tool?
Routine clinical range of motion measurements are often done very cursorily or relegated to ancillary medical personnel, with use of estimation rather than proper instrumentation and standardized technique. In the defense of most clinicians, it may be argued that routine range of motion measurements are performed to objectify symptoms and assess clinical progress, and hence do not justify the investment of a lot of time or effort for accuracy.

Numerous factors affect range of motion and the analysis of all parts of "the examiner, the examined and the examination" are essential [2]. As with any other scientific measurement, range of motion measurements should be reliable and valid. This requires measurement and documentation methods to be standardized, so that measurements are accurate, reliable, and comparable.

Historically, the spinal range of motion measurements have progressed from visual estimation to the use of goniometers and inclinometers and subsequently to more complex measurement tools involving computer-assisted video motion analysis. The gain in accuracy, and to some extent reliability, of the increasingly complex methods is offset by the time taken for the measurement and the lack of portability of the instruments.

Types

Visual estimation

The usefulness of visual estimation of range of motion has been controversial. Although some earlier studies have suggested that visual estimation is as good as or better than goniometric measurement [3, 4], this has not been upheld by more recent studies [5–7]. Studies by Nelson et al [8] and Rae et al [9] demonstrated that measurements varied by as much as 30% with the use of the single observational method of Hoppenfeld [10]. This high degree of variability makes visual estimation an unsatisfactory method of measurement. Measurement with instruments is preferable when accuracy and reliability are essential.

Goniometer

The two-arm goniometer is the instrument most widely used by clinicians to measure range of motion. It is economical, portable and well evaluated in many studies [7, 12]. Accurate measurement of the often complex and compound motions of the spine are rendered difficult with a conventional goniometer. A variety of modifications of the goniometer have been devised to overcome these practical difficulties [11]. These include the inclinometer, which comes in mechanical or electronic form. The ability of the inclinometer to measure spinal movements with accuracy and reliability is well documented for both lumbar and cervical spinal movements [12, 14].

Computer-assisted video motion analysis

Computer-assisted video motion analysis (optoelectronic) systems and infrared 3-D systems have been used for range of motion determination in the spine. The advantage of these systems is the ability to study the nature of complex motions of the spine and the relationship of intersegmental spinal motion. The limitation of these systems is the variability of the application and reapplications of the skin markers and the individual variability in the movement of the skin at the point of application of the markers [13].

Cervical spine

Most cervical movements are a combination of more than one of the following basic motions:

- Flexion/extension
- Lateral bending
- Rotation

Thus, testing pure flexion/extension, lateral bending, and rotation is very difficult. However, approximately 50% flexion/extension occurs between the occiput (C0) and C1 with the remaining 50% distributed in the subaxial spine (maximally at C5/6). Lateral bending is actually not a pure motion but a combination of rotation and translation. Maximal contribution is in the upper part of subaxial region (C2/3 and C3/4). It is well known that 50% of rotation occurs between C1 and C2 because of their special anatomy and the remaining 50% is distributed in the subaxial region (maximally at C5/6).

Flexion/extension

Active: Instruct the patient to roll his head forward so that he is able to touch his chin to his chest if he has a normal flexion. The chin-chest distance can be measured for recording purposes. Ask him to look at the ceiling above to judge his extension. The patient should be seated and erect. The plane of the nose and forehead should be nearly horizontal if he has a normal extension. The arc of motion should be watched carefully because it is usually smooth. Painful conditions may not only limit range of motion but also make the act of motion hesitant or jittery.

Passive: For passive tests of neck flexion/extension, the clinician's hand should be placed to either side of the patient's cranium and the head is tilted forwards or backwards maximally.

How to measure: A spatula may be held in the mouth and a goni-ometer may be used for measuring normal range about flexion 80° and extension 50°.

Lateral bending—left/right
Active: Ask the patient to tilt his head and touch his ear to his shoulder without allowing him to lift his shoulder. This ma-neuver is judged from the front and the back of the patient.

Passive: The clinician holds the lateral aspect of the patient's head with one hand and stabilizes the ipsilateral shoulder with the other. The head is then rolled on to the sides in an at-tempt to touch the shoulder. The movement is repeated on the other side after changing over the hands. In torticollis due to sternomastoid contracture, the muscles stand out when lateral bending to the opposite side is tested. Attempted passive lateral bending in extension may produce a sharp shooting pain on one side (Spurling's test) and is said to be diagnostic of cervical disc prolapse presenting with radiculopathy.

How to measure: A spatula that is held in the mouth may be used for recording purposes. Normal range is about 45° on either side.

Rotation—left/right:
Active: Ask the patient to look over his shoulder. He should be able to move his head so that the chin just falls short of the plane of the shoulders. Torticollis on one side frequently lim-its the opposite rotation. Rotation is frequently restricted and painful in degenerative conditions of the cervical spine.

Passive: The examiner should be standing behind the patient and place one hand on the patient's chin. The other hand should stabilize the patient's shoulder while the chin is rotated to the other side.

How to measure: A spatula that is held in the mouth may be used as a pointer for recording purposes. Normal range is about 80° on either side.

Thoracolumbar spine

In absence of restraining ribs in the lumbar spine, more flexion/extension can take place in the lumbar spine than in the thoracic spine. Major flexion primarily involves motion in the hip and hence, even in long segment fusion of the thoracolumbar spine, the patient's ability to bend forwards and backwards remains mostly unaffected. However, due to the near anteroposterior orientation of the lumbar facets as opposed to the near mediolateral orientation of the thoracic facets, rotation mostly occurs in the thoracic spine. Lateral bending has almost equal contributions on the thoracic and lumbar spine. It is important to realize that it is extremely difficult to exactly segregate the contributions of all these movements by the thoracic/lumbar spine and hence they are considered together as the thoracolumbar spine.

Flexion/extension

Active: Ask the patient to bend forward as far as he can to try and touch his toes with the knees straight. The distance from the fingertips to the ground gives a reasonable idea of the amount of flexion and can be measured. The majority of patients can reach the floor or within 7 cm from it. Of course, this does not indicate the relative contributions of the hip and spine. For testing extension, ask the patient to arch his back as much as possible.

Passive: Stand by the side of the patient and place one hand on the upper back and the other on the lower abdomen, gently bending the subject forwards. The hand on the back at the terminal range should exert mild pressure. For measuring passive extension, stand beside the patient and place one hand on the back (to steady the pelvis) and pull back the shoulder with the other hand as much as possible.

How to measure: Besides measuring the distance of the fingertip to the floor with a tape measure, we can measure the increase in interspinous distance as the patient bends forwards. This is more appreciable in the lumbar spine than in the thoracic spine and excludes hip motion. An extension of this method is Schober's Test in which a 10 cm length of lumbar spine is used as a base. We begin by vertically holding the tape in the midline of the lumbar spine so that the 10 cm mark is at the level of the posterior superior iliac spine (dimples of Venus/small of the back). Then mark the skin at the 0 cm and 15 cm mark, anchor the top of the tape with a finger and ask the patient to bend forward. Note the tape measure at the 15 cm skin mark when the patient fully bends forward. Normally, there should be an increment of about 6–7 cm; less than 5 cm is indicative of spinal pathology. This method can be extrapolated to the thoracic spine with the upper point at the nape of the neck 30 cm from the previous 0 mark. Note the increase as the patient bends forward. This is normally about 3 cm. To measure extension, the decrease in distance between L1 and S1 on extension may be measured with a tape. Measurement of flexion and extension by a goniometer is difficult.

Lateral bending

Active: Ask the patient to slide the hands down the side of each thigh. It is good practice to stabilize the patient while this is being done.

Passive: Stabilize the patient's pelvis with one hand, grip the opposite shoulder with the other and make him lean to the same side.

How to measure: One can measure the distance between the tip of the finger and the floor with a tape as in flexion. Alternatively, the angle between the vertical and a line drawn through the spinous processes of T1 to S1 can be measured with a goniometer. It is about 30° on either side with equal contribution to the thoracic and lumbar spine.

Rotation

Active: Once the patient has been seated, ask him to twist around to each side. Sitting ensures stabilization of the pelvis.

Passive: The examiner stands behind the patient with one hand on his iliac crest to stabilize the pelvis. The other hand is placed on the opposite shoulder, which is turned posteriorly to the maximum. The same procedure is repeated for the opposite side after switching the position of the hands.

How to measure: Rotation is measured between the plane of the shoulders and the pelvis, which is usually taken to be neutral. Normal range is about 40° on either side; most of it being contributed to by the thoracic spine.

Summary

Motion of the spine is an interesting phenomenon, frequently used as a substitute for measuring spinal function or even health. Although spinal motion is easily measured, its contribution to the global spinal health assessment is not yet fully understood. Perhaps a multimodality motion measurement incorporating strength and pain reproduction may enhance our future understanding of spinal motion.

References

1. **Hart DL, Berlin S, Brager PE, et al** (1994) Development of clinical standards in industrial rehabilitation. *J Orthop Sports Phys Ther;* 19:232–241.

2. **Stratford P, Agostino V, Brazeau C, et al** (1984) Reliability of joint angle measurement: a discussion of methodology issues. *Physiother Canada;* 36:5–9.

3. **American Academy of Orthopaedic Surgeons** (1965) *Joint Motion: Method of Measuring and Recording.* American Academy of Orthopaedic Surgeons: Chicago.

4. **Rowe CR** (1964) Joint measurement in disability evaluation. *Clin Orthop Relat Res;* 32:43–53.

5. **Hoppenbrouwers M, Eckhardt MM, Verkerk K, et al** (2006) Reproducibility of the measurement of active and passive cervical range of motion. *J Manipulative Physiol Ther;* 29:363–367.

6. **Viikari-Juntura E** (1987) Interexaminer reliability of observations in physical examinations of the neck. *Phys Ther;* 67:1526–1532.

7. **Youdas JW, Carey JR, Garrett TR** (1991) Reliability of measurements of cervical spine range of motion—comparison of three methods. *Phys Ther;* 71:98–104; discussion 105–106.

8. **Nelson MA, Allen P, Clamp SE, et al** (1979) Reliability and reproducibility of clinical findings in low-back pain. *Spine (Phila Pa 1976);* 4:97–101.

9. **Rae PS, Waddell G, Venner RM** (1984) A simple technique for measuring lumbar spinal flexion. Its use in orthopaedic practice. *J R Coll Surg Edinb;* 29:281–284.

10. **Hoppenfeld S** (1976) *Physical Examination of the Spine and Extremities.* Appleton-Centuri-Crofts: New York.

11. **Agarwal S, Allison GT, Singer KP** (2005) Reliability of the spin-t cervical goniometer in measuring cervical range of motion in an asymptomatic indian population. *J Manipulative Physiol Ther* 2005; 28:487–492.

12. **Yankai A, Manosan P** (2009) Reliability of the Universal and Invented Gravity Goniometers in Measuring Active Cervical Range of Motion in Normal Healthy Subjects. *International Journal of applied biomedical engineering* vol.2, no.1, 49–53.

13. **Jordan K, Dziedzic K, Mullis R, et al** (2001) The development of three-dimensional range of motion measurement systems for clinical practice. *Rheuymatology;* 40:1081–88.

14. **Kachingwe AF, Phillips BJ** (2005) Inter- and Intrarater Reliability of a Back Range of Motion Instrument. *Arch Phys Med Rehabil;* 86:2347–2352.

3.1.1   Types

---

1   Visual estimation

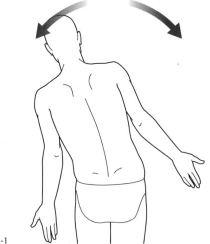

Fig 3.1.1-1

Description
Measuring passive or active range of motion by visual estimation only, without a measuring device.

Interpretation
A qualitative assessment that is based clinical examination.

Clinical relevance
As this is a largely qualitative analysis, it is difficult to use visual estimation against population standards. However, it can be useful when evaluating serial measurements within the same patient.

SCORING   *10 total points*

Scientific   *5 points*

○ Interobserver reliability
○ Intraobserver reliability
● Universality
○● Disease specificity

Clinical utility   *5 points*

● Ease of application
● Simplicity
● Patient tolerability
●● Affordability

●●●●●●●○○○   **7**

Reliability

Population tested in	Interobserver reliability	Intraobserver reliability
Neck and radicular pain patients (N = 52) were evaluated by a physical medicine and rehabilitation physician and a physical therapist [1]	-	-
Patients with orthopaedic disorders of the cervical spine (N = 60) were evaluated twice within the same day by eleven volunteer physical therapists with clinical experience ranging from 2 to 27 years [2]	-	-

References:
1. Viikari-Juntura E (1987) Interexaminer reliability of observations in physical examinations of the neck. *Phys Ther;* 67:1526–1532.
2. Youdas JW, Carey JR, Garrett TR (1991) Reliability of measurements of cervical spine range of motion–comparison of three methods. *Phys Ther;* 71:98–104; discussion 105–106.

2 Goniometer

Description
An instrument used to measure joint angles.

Interpretation
Goniometers can be used to assess range of motion prior to an intervention, and then used again to assess range of motion after intervention to determine success.

Clinical relevance
Though there is some inherent intraobserver and interobserver variability, this is a more quantitative assessment than simple visual estimation.

References:
1. Cleland JA, Childs JD, Fritz JM, et al (2006) Interrater reliability of the history and physical examination in patients with mechanical neck pain. *Arch Phys Med Rehabil;* 87:1388–1395.
2. Maksymowych WP, Mallon C, Richardson R, et al (2006) Development and validation of a simple tape-based measurement tool for recording cervical rotation in patients with ankylosing spondylitis: comparison with a goniometer-based approach. *J Rheumatol;* 33:2242–2249.
3. Pellecchia GL, Bohannon RW (1998) Active lateral neck flexion range of motion measurements obtained with a modified goniometer: reliability and estimates of normal. *J Manipulative Physiol Ther;* 21:443–447.
4. Youdas JW, Carey JR, Garrett TR (1991) Reliability of measurements of cervical spine range of motion–comparison of three methods. *Phys Ther;* 71:98-104; discussion 105–106.
5. Nitschke JE, Nattrass CL, Disler PB, et al (1999) Reliability of the American Medical Association guides' model for measuring spinal range of motion. Its implication for whole-person impairment rating. *Spine (Phila Pa 1976);* 24:262–268.

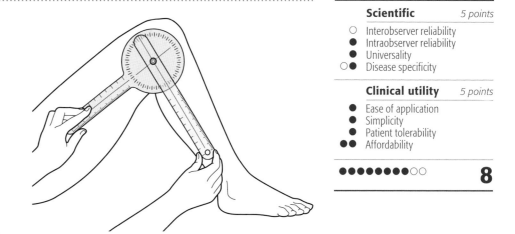

Fig 3.1.1-2

SCORING *10 total points*

Scientific *5 points*
○ Interobserver reliability
● Intraobserver reliability
● Universality
○● Disease specificity

Clinical utility *5 points*
● Ease of application
● Simplicity
● Patient tolerability
●● Affordability

●●●●●●●●○○ **8**

Reliability

Population tested in	Interobserver reliability	Intraobserver reliability
Mechanical neck pain patients (N = 22) were evaluated by four physical therapists using a universal goniometer [1]	-	NA
Patients with anklyosing spondylitis (N = 44) were evaluated by a clinician nurse, rheumatologist, and trained medical student [2]	+	+
Healthy subjects (N = 100) were tested using a plastic goniometer by two physical therapists with 13 and 2 years experience [3]	-	+
Patients with orthopaedic disorders of the cervical spine (N = 60) were evaluated twice within the same day by eleven volunteer physical therapists with clinical experience ranging from 2–27 years [4]	-	+
Chronic low back pain patients (N = 34) were evaluated with a long-arm goniometer on two occasions 2 weeks apart by two observers [5]	-	-
A systematic review evaluating cervical ROM, single inclinometer, and EDI 320 in patients with non-specific neck pain	+	+

3   Computer-assisted video motion analysis (optoelectronic) systems

SCORING   *10 total points*

Description
Patient is videotaped performing various motions. Computer software is then used to analyze motion.

Some systems use skin markers placed on specific anatomical landmarks. For example, for flexion and extension of the lumbar spine markers are placed at the sternum, at T1, T12, and S2, at the greater trochanter, and 5–10 cm below the greater trochanter.

Interpretation
Once marker identification is confirmed, the software program automatically analyzes and computes range of motion.

Clinical relevance
Useful test for gait analysis that may also have a role in deformity assessment.

The advantage is the ability to study the nature of complex motions of the spine and the relationship of intersegmental spinal motion.

The limitation is the variability of the application and reapplications of the skin markers and the individual variability in the movement of the skin at the point of application of the markers.

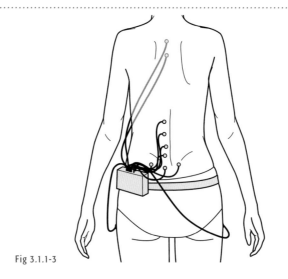

Fig 3.1.1-3

Scientific   *5 points*

○ Interobserver reliability
○ Intraobserver reliability
● Universality
○● Disease specificity

Clinical utility   *5 points*

○ Ease of application
○ Simplicity
● Patient tolerability
○● Affordability

●●●●○○○○○○   **4**

Reliability

Population tested in	Interobserver reliability	Intraobserver reliability
Not tested		

4 Infrared 3-D systems

Description
Two or more sets of reflective marker clusters are placed at specific anatomical landmarks. An anatomical coordinate system is linked to the thorax using 3-D coordinates.

Interpretation
The 3-D shape of the spine and the segmental rotations of the cervical, thoracic, and lumbar spine can be captured.

Clinical relevance
The advantage is the ability to study the nature of complex motions of the spine and the relationship of intersegmental spinal motion.

The limitation is the variability of the application and reapplications of the skin markers and the individual variability in the movement of the skin at the point of application of the markers.

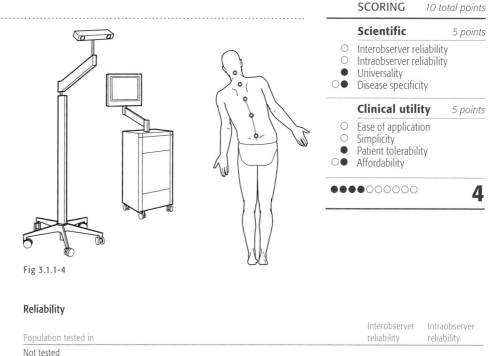

Fig 3.1.1-4

SCORING   *10 total points*

Scientific   *5 points*
○ Interobserver reliability
○ Intraobserver reliability
● Universality
○● Disease specificity

Clinical utility   *5 points*
○ Ease of application
○ Simplicity
● Patient tolerability
○● Affordability

●●●●○○○○○○   **4**

Reliability

Population tested in	Interobserver reliability	Intraobserver reliability
Not tested		

3.1.2   Cervical spine-specific

1   Flexion/extension

Description
Active: Patient moves head forward (chin to chest) to measure flexion.

Patient looks to the ceiling above to measure extension.

A spatula may be held in patient's mouth and goniometer used for measuring range of motion.

Interpretation
Approximate normal range:
- Flexion 80°
- Extension 50°

Clinical relevance
While there is variability between patients and user measurements, this method provides a general assessment of overall motion.
Absolute values of motion can be compared against the average range of the general population.
However, these measurements can also be used to compare serial measurements in the same individual.

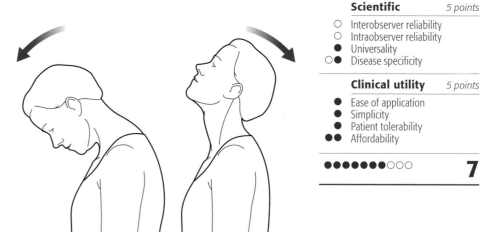

Fig 3.1.2-1

Scientific   *5 points*
- ○ Interobserver reliability
- ○ Intraobserver reliability
- ● Universality
- ○● Disease specificity

Clinical utility   *5 points*
- ● Ease of application
- ● Simplicity
- ● Patient tolerability
- ●● Affordability

●●●●●●●○○○   **7**

Reliability

Population tested in	Interobserver reliability	Intraobserver reliability
Not tested		

2 Lateral bending

Description

Active: Patient is asked to touch the left ear to the left shoulder. This is repeated with the right ear to the right shoulder.

This motion is to be done without allowing the patient to lift the shoulder.

A spatula may be held in the mouth for recording purposes.

Interpretation

Approximate normal range:
• Either side 45°

Clinical relevance

While there is variability between patients and user measurements, this method provides a general assessment of overall motion.
Absolute values of motion can be compared against the average range of the general population.
However, these measurements can also be used to compare serial measurements in the same individual.

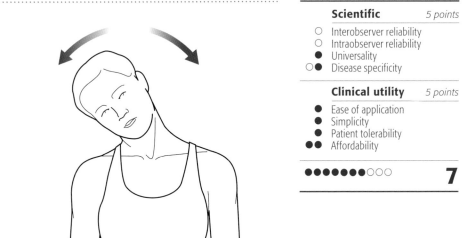

Fig 3.1.2-2

SCORING	10 total points

Scientific	5 points
○	Interobserver reliability
○	Intraobserver reliability
●	Universality
○●	Disease specificity

Clinical utility	5 points
●	Ease of application
●	Simplicity
●	Patient tolerability
●●	Affordability

●●●●●●●○○○ **7**

Reliability

Population tested in	Interobserver reliability	Intraobserver reliability
Not tested		

3   Rotation

Description
Patient is instructed to look over the shoulder, and should be able to move his head so that the chin falls just short of the plane of the shoulders.

Torticollis on one side frequently limits the opposite rotation. Rotation is frequently restricted and painful in degenerative conditions of the cervical spine.

A spatula may be held in the mouth for recording purposes.

Interpretation
Approximate normal range:
• Either side 80°

Clinical relevance
While there is variability between patients and user measurements, this method provides a general assessment of overall motion.
Absolute values of motion can be compared against the average range of the general population.
However, these measurements can also be used to compare serial measurements in the same individual.

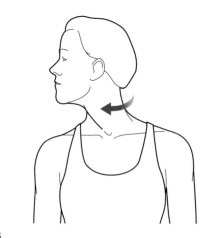

Fig 3.1.2-3

SCORING   *10 total points*

Scientific   *5 points*
○ Interobserver reliability
○ Intraobserver reliability
● Universality
○● Disease specificity

Clinical utility   *5 points*
● Ease of application
● Simplicity
● Patient tolerability
●● Affordability

●●●●●●●○○○   **7**

Reliability

Population tested in	Interobserver reliability	Intraobserver reliability
Not tested		

3.1.3 Thoracolumbar spine-specific

1 Flexion/extension

Description

Active: In order to measure flexion, the patient bends forward in an attempt to touch his toes while keeping the knees straight. The distance from the fingertips to the ground gives a reasonable idea of the amount of flexion and can be measured as well. This does not indicate the relative contributions of the hip and spine.

For testing extension the patient arches their back as much as possible.

Interpretation

The majority of patients can reach the floor or within 7 cm from it.

Clinical relevance

While there is variability between patients, this method provides a general assessment of overall motion. Absolute values of motion can be compared against the average range of the general population. However, this measurement can also be used to compare serial measurements in the same individual.

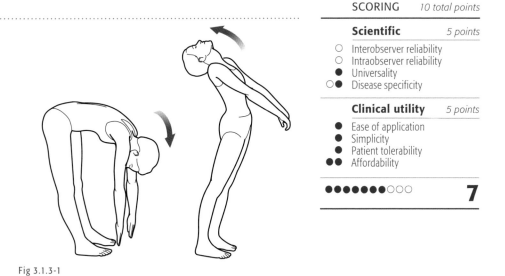

Fig 3.1.3-1

SCORING	10 total points
Scientific	5 points
○ Interobserver reliability	
○ Intraobserver reliability	
● Universality	
○● Disease specificity	
Clinical utility	5 points
● Ease of application	
● Simplicity	
● Patient tolerability	
●● Affordability	

●●●●●●●○○○   **7**

Reliability

Population tested in	Interobserver reliability	Intraobserver reliability
Not tested		

2   Schober's Test [1]

Description
A 10 cm length of lumbar spine is used as a base. The tape is held vertically in the midline of the lumbar spine so that the 10 cm mark is at the level of the posterior superior iliac spine (dimples of Venus/small of the back). The skin is marked at the 0 cm and 15 cm mark, the top of the tape is anchored with a finger, and the patient bends forward.

To measure extension, the decrease in distance between L1 and S1 on extension may be measured with a tape. Measurement of flexion and extension by a goniometer is difficult.

Interpretation
Note the tape measure at the 15 cm skin mark when the patient fully bends forward. Normally, there should be an increment of about 6–7 cm. Less than 5 cm is indicative of spinal pathology.

Clinical relevance
This provides a general assessment of spinal mobility.

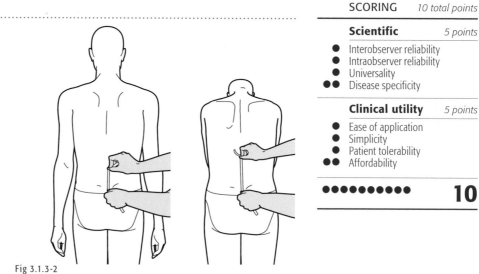

Fig 3.1.3-2

SCORING	10 total points
Scientific	5 points

- Interobserver reliability
- Intraobserver reliability
- Universality
- ●● Disease specificity

Clinical utility	5 points

- Ease of application
- Simplicity
- Patient tolerability
- ●● Affordability

●●●●●●●●●●   **10**

Reliability

Population tested in	Interobserver reliability	Intraobserver reliability
Patients with idiopathic ankylosing spondylitis (N = 54) were evaluated using the modified Schober's Test by five physical therapists [2]	+	+
Low back pain patients (N = 31) were evaluated using the Modified-Modified Schober's Test by two independent observers [3]	+	+

References:
1. Schober P (1937) Lendenwirbelsaule und Kreuzschmerzen. *Much Med Wochenschr;* 84:336–339. German.
2. Viitanen JV, Kokko ML, Heikkila S, et al (1999) Assessment of thoracolumbar rotation in ankylosing spondylitis: a simple tape method. *Clin Rheumatol;* 18:152–157.
3. Tousignant M, Poulin L, Marchand S, et al (2005) The Modified-Modified Schober Test for range of motion assessment of lumbar flexion in patients with low back pain: a study of criterion validity, intra- and inter-rater reliability and minimum metrically detectable change. *Disabil Rehabil;* 27:553–559.

3   Lateral bending

Description
Active: Patient slides his left hand down
the side of the left thigh.
This is repeated with the right hand
down the side of the right thigh.
The patient should be stabilized
throughout.

Interpretation
One can measure the distance between
the tip of the finger and the floor with
a tape.

Alternatively, the angle between the
vertical line and a line drawn through
the spinous processes of T1 to S1 can
be measured with a goniometer.
It is about 30° on either side with equal
contribution to the thoracic and
lumbar spine.

Clinical relevance
While there is variability between
patients, this method provides a
general assessment of overall motion.
Absolute values of motion can be
compared against the average range of
the general population. However, this
measurement can also be used to
compare serial measurements in the
same individual.

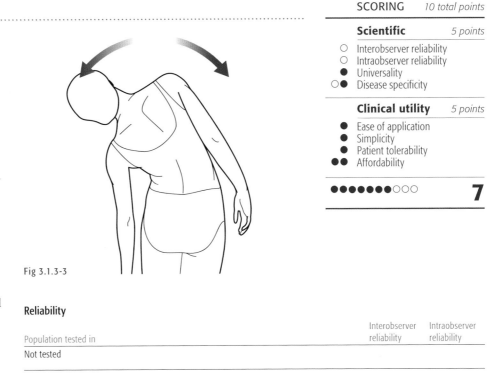

Fig 3.1.3-3

Reliability

Population tested in	Interobserver reliability	Intraobserver reliability
Not tested		

4   Rotation

Description

Active: Patient has to be seated and is asked to twist around to each side. Sitting ensures stabilization of the pelvis.

Interpretation

Rotation is measured between the plane of the shoulders and the pelvis.

Normal range is about 40° on either side, most of it being contributed by the thoracic spine.

Clinical relevance

This measurement provides a general assessment of patient motion. Care must be taken to ensure the pelvis remains neutral so as not to inadvertently overestimate rotatory motion.

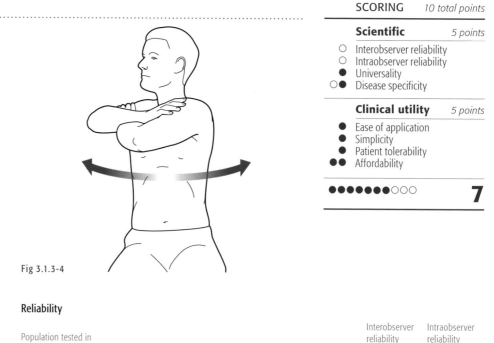

Fig 3.1.3-4

Reliability

Population tested in	Interobserver reliability	Intraobserver reliability
Not tested		

SCORING   *10 total points*

Scientific   *5 points*

○ Interobserver reliability
○ Intraobserver reliability
● Universality
○● Disease specificity

Clinical utility   *5 points*

● Ease of application
● Simplicity
● Patient tolerability
●● Affordability

●●●●●●●○○○   **7**

3   Clinical measurements
3.2 Neurological measurements

3 Clinical measurements

3.2 Neurological measurements

Introduction

....

Spinal examination allows for localization of spinal cord pathology along the rostrocaudal axis and the transverse plane. It creates an objective correlation between clinical deficits and radiographic findings, thereby helping to predict the necessity and benefit of surgical intervention. A careful observation of the patterns of deficits will also allow for discrimination between true spinal pathology and nonneurological disease. In this chapter we will discuss measurements of function on the spinal examination. We will explore current clinical scores and scales of spinal disease, focusing specifically on quantifiable tests of motor and sensory performance, reflexes and complex function. An overview of these tests can be found in **Table 3.2-1.**

Category	Tests
Motor	Medical Research Council (MRC) Grading System
	Hand-held dynamometer
	Wolf motor function test (WMF)
	Jebson-Taylor hand function test (JTHF)
	Nine-hole peg test
	Graded and redefined assessment of strength, sensibility and prehension (GRASSP)
Sensory	American Spinal Injury Association (ASIA) impairment scale — sensory
	Quantitative sensory testing
Tone and reflexes	National Institute of Neurological Disorders and Stroke (NINDS) myotactic reflex scale
	Ashworth scale
Autonomic	ASIA impairment scale—autonomic
Walking	10-meter walk test (10MWT)
	30-meter walk test (30MWT)
	50-foot walk test (50FWT)
	Timed up and go test (TUG)
	10-second step test (10SST)
	Washington index for spinal injury (WISC-II)
	Spinal cord injury functional ambulation inventory (SCI-FAE)
Composite scales	ASIA/International Medical Society of Paraplegia (IMSOP)
	Functional independence measure (FIM)
	Spinal cord independence measure (SCIM)
	Rivermead mobility index (RMI)
	Barthel index
	Fugl-Meyer assessment
	Quadriplegia index of function (QIF)

Table 3.2-1 Overview of quantitative tests in spinal examination.

Motor

The Medical Research Council grading system

The most widely used measurement of motor strength is the Medical Research Council (MRC) muscle strength grading system. The MRC grading system is a 5-point ordinal scale ranging from 0 (no visible muscle contraction) to 5 (full strength). Its origins date back to World War II, when the Nerve Injuries Committee of the British Army published Aids to the Investigation of Peripheral Nerve Injuries [1] in the hope of creating a quantifiable grading scale to measure recovery in patients with traumatic nerve injuries resulting in paralysis. Since its first publication in 1943, the MRC grading system has attracted considerable debate. While it is supported by reasonable interobserver and intraobserver reliability [2], it is heavily reliant on a limb's ability to perform against gravity and the percentage of total strength required to raise a limb against gravity, which varies between muscle groups [3]. In electrophysiological studies, the brachii muscle requires ~2% of total strength to raise the forearm against gravity, hip abductor muscles require 24%, and supinator muscles require < 1% [4]. Similarly, cadaveric studies have shown that total torque required to flex the elbow against gravity is as low as 4% [5]. Therefore the single grade 4/5 represented more than 96% of total functional ability. Bearing in mind that the original intention of the MRC grading system was to track subtle improvements in patients with post-traumatic paralysis, it is reasonable that the scale is heavily biased towards small, objective improvements in motor function (grades 0–3) with disproportionally large jumps between high strength grades (grades 4–5). However, when used in the context of degenerative disc disease where patients typically retain near-full strength, the 5-point grading system becomes less objective and more reliant on the subjective proprioception of the examiner. While many other functional manual motor tests (MMTs) exist and will be addressed later, the MRC grading system remains the dominant scale in assessing motor function for its simplicity. It has also been incorporated into many of the composite grading systems. The American Spinal Injury Association (ASIA)/International Medical Society of Paraplegia (IMSOP) impairment scale is a multifaceted classification system of spinal cord injury that has been adopted by many physicians who manage acute spinal cord injury. The motor arm of the scale incorporates the MRC grading system for testing muscle strength. The algorithm used to calculate the ASIA score can be found in **Fig 3.2-1a–b**. In combination with sensory examination, the level and lateralization of the MRC grade is used to determine the single neurological level (the lowest segment where motor and sensory function is normal, on both sides, and the most cranial of the sensory and motor levels). The ASIA/IMSOP impairment scale will be discussed in greater detail later.

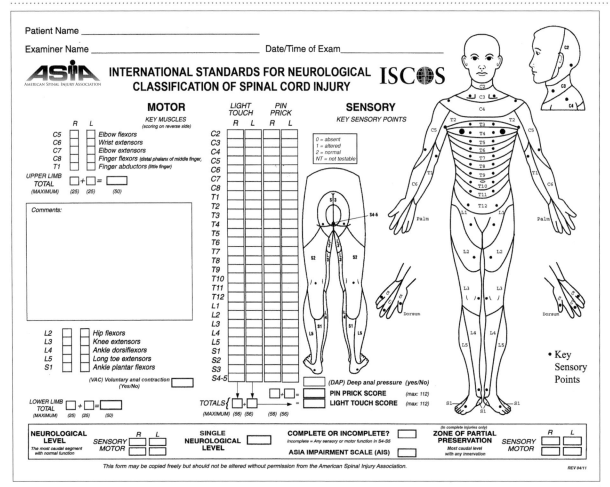

Fig 3.2-1a–b American Spinal Injury Association: International Standards for Neurological Classification of Spinal Cord Injury, revised 2011; Atlanta, GA. Reprinted 2011.
a Standard neurological classification of spinal cord injury with sensory and motor examination

Muscle Function Grading

0 = total paralysis

1 = palpable or visible contraction

2 = active movement, full range of motion (ROM) with gravity eliminated

3 = active movement, full ROM against gravity

4 = active movement, full ROM against gravity and moderate resistance in a muscle specific position.

5 = (normal) active movement, full ROM against gravity and full resistance in a muscle specific position expected from an otherwise unimpaired peson.

5* = (normal) active movement, full ROM against gravity and sufficient resistance to be considered normal if identified inhibiting factors (i.e. pain, disuse) were not present.

NT = not testable (i.e. due to immobilization, severe pain such that the patient cannot be graded, amputation of limb, or contracture of >50% of the range of motion).

ASIA Impairment (AIS) Scale

☐ **A = Complete.** No sensory or motor function is preserved in the sacral segments S4-S5.

☐ **B = Sensory Incomplete.** Sensory but not motor function is preserved below the neurological level and includes the sacral segments S4-S5 (light touch, pin prick at S4-S5: or deep anal pressure (DAP)), AND no motor function is preserved more than three levels below the motor level on either side of the body.

☐ **C = Motor Incomplete.** Motor function is preserved below the neurological level**, and more than half of key muscle functions below the single neurological level of injury (NLI) have a muscle grade less than 3 (Grades 0-2).

☐ **D = Motor Incomplete.** Motor function is preserved below the neurological level**, and at least half (half or more) of key muscle functions below the NLI have a muscle grade ≥ 3.

☐ **E = Normal.** If sensation and motor function as tested with the ISNCSCI are graded as normal in all segments, and the patient had prior deficits, then the AIS grade is E. Someone without an initial SCI does not receive an AIS grade.

**For an individual to receive a grade of C or D, i.e. motor incomplete status, they must have either (1) voluntary anal sphincter contraction or (2) sacral sensory sparing with sparing of motor function more than three levels below the motor level for that side of the body. The Standards at this time allows even non-key muscle function more than 3 levels below the motor level to be used in determining motor incomplete status (AIS B versus C).

NOTE: When assessing the extent of motor sparing below the level for distinguishing between AIS B and C, the *motor level* on each side is used; whereas to differentiate between AIS C and D (based on proportion of key muscle functions with strength grade 3 or greater) the *single neurological level* is used.

Steps in Classification

The following order is recommended in determining the classification of individuals with SCI.

1. Determine sensory levels for right and left sides.

2. Determine motor levels for right and left sides.
   Note: in regions where there is no myotome to test, the motor level is presumed to be the same as the sensory level, if testable motor function above that level is also normal.

3. Determine the single neurological level.
   This is the lowest segment where motor and sensory function is normal on both sides, and is the most cephalad of the sensory and motor levels determined in steps 1 and 2.

4. Determine whether the injury is Complete or Incomplete.
   (i.e. absence or presence of sacral sparing)
   If voluntary anal contraction = No AND all S4-5 sensory scores = 0 AND deep anal pressure = No, then injury is COMPLETE. Otherwise, injury is incomplete.

5. Determine ASIA Impairment Scale (AIS) Grade:
   Is injury Complete?   If **YES**, AIS=A and can record ZPP
   (lowest dermatome or myotome on each side with some preservation)

   NO

   Is injury motor Incomplete?   If **NO**, AIS=B
   (Yes=voluntary anal contraction OR motor function more than three levels below the motor level on a given side, if the patient has sensory incomplete classification)

   YES

   Are at least half of the key muscles below the single neurological level graded 3 or better?

   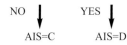

   NO → AIS=C   YES → AIS=D

   If sensation and motor function is normal in all segments, AIS=E
   Note: AIS E is used in follow-up testing when an individual with a documented SCI has recovered normal function. If at initial testing no deficits are found, the individual is neurologically intact; the ASIA Impairment Scale does not apply.

Fig 3.2-1a–b (cont.) American Spinal Injury Association: International Standards for Neurological Classification of Spinal Cord Injury, revised 2011; Atlanta, GA. Reprinted 2011.
b Instructions and classification information

Quantified muscle tests

Efforts have been made to create quantified muscle tests (QMTs) to allow for concrete measurements of muscle function, particularly in clinical research. QMTs use dynamometric equipment to get an absolute measurement, in kilograms or newtons, of a muscle groups' strength. Unfortunately, they often require bulky equipment and are heavily reliant on the technician's skill. They have been criticized for a lack of standardized clinical relevance. While a value given in MMT scales reflect the functional ability of a patient (ie, for a limb to overcome gravity), the value at which a dynamometric measurement implies clinical change is poorly defined (ie, at what value can a patient feed themselves). Nonetheless, the hand-held dynamometer is a portable and objective tool that shows promise of becoming a simple and concrete method of following rehabilitation or disease progression.

Upper extremity testing

The motor performance of the hand has unique implications in quality of life. The Wolf motor function test (WMF), the Jebson-Taylor hand function test (JTHF), and the 9-hole peg test are tests specifically focused on the complex function of the upper extremity. The WMF and JTHF both test commonly performed manual tasks (ie, writing, reading, feeding, and manipulating objects). While the JTHF is scored based on time required to complete each task, the WMF has both timed and force-based components that are further scored on quality of movement. The 9-hole peg test is a timed examination wherein the patient places and then removes dowels from nine set holes. While the WMF and JTHF are appropriately detailed for a research setting, the nine-hole peg test provides a convenient and easily reproducible test of fine motor skill that may be more applicable to the clinical setting. The graded and redefined assessment of strength, sensibility and prehension (GRASSP) is a battery of tests quantifying upper extremity function [6].

Sensory

There are few sensory grading scales for spinal cord injury. The ASIA impairment scale incorporates a sum score for all dermatomes that are measured using light touch and pin prick [7]. The ASIA impairment scale can be found in **Fig 3.2-1b**. The score is 0 for no sensation, 1 for reduced sensation, and 2 for normal sensation. Some studies have utilized computer-controlled psychophysics experiments using cold and vibration for a more detailed assessment of sensory loss [8]. Although more detailed, these techniques require equipment that is not widely available in the clinical setting. Other clinically important tests, such as the proprioception test, are difficult to quantify, but generally could be present, reduced, or absent.

Tone and reflexes

Traditionally, scales used to measure deep tendon reflexes have been varied with poor standardization between centers and significant interrater variability. However, Hallett et al [9] introduced a myotactic reflex scale that was clearly defined and found to have improved interobserver reliability and excellent intraobserver reliability [10]. The National Institute of Neurological Disorders and Stroke (NINDS) myotactic reflex scale is now widely accepted as the standard of measurement of deep tendon reflexes. It is a 5-point scale that ranges from 0, indicating no reflex, to 4+, indicating more than normal with or without clonus. Though shown to have improved validity over past scales and good reliability when used by trained specialists [10], the NINDS scale has poor reliability when used in the day-to-day practice of physicians of different specialties and training [11]. Nonetheless, this scale has, for the most part, taken over the previously popular Mayo Clinic scale for tendon reflex assessment [12]. Its main advantage is simplicity. The Mayo Clinic scale ranges from -4 to +4 with subtle differences between largely subjective points (-3 for Just elicitable, -2 for Low, -1 for Moderately low), while the NINDS scale presents only 5, more distinct scoring options.

The degree of spasticity can change depending on the time of day, level of activity, ambient temperature, and even emotional status [13]. Because of this, it is particularly difficult to create reliable scales of spasticity. The Ashworth and modified Ashworth scale are the best supported scoring systems for spasticity. First published in 1964 and then modified by Bohannon and Smith in 1987, the Ashworth scale measures tone and rigidity in a 5-point ordinal scale ranging from no increase in tone to rigid in flexion or extension [14]. It has high interrater variability, which is somewhat better in the upper extremity than in the lower extremity [15]. Electrophysiological and biomechanical techniques have been helpful in creating quantitative measurements of resistance, and have pro-

vided insight into the pathophysiology of spasticity. However, to date they have been shown to have limited clinical use and a simple, portable instrument has not yet been developed [16].

The Hoffman and Babinski signs are reliable tests for spasticity and myelopathy [17]. Genital reflexes, including the bulbocavernosus and cremasteric reflexes, are commonly used to assess spinal shock. As these reflexes are either present or absent they are not typically quantified.

Assessment of the autonomic nervous system

Recently, a consensus panel convened by ASIA has codified a series of objective tests to quantitate changes in the autonomic nervous system [18]. These tests can be found in **Fig 3.2-2** and include the cardiovascular, temperature regulation, genito-urinary, and gastrointestinal systems, given the impact that spinal disease and injury can have on this aspect of nervous system function.

AUTONOMIC STANDARDS ASSESSMENT FORM
Patient Name: _____

Anatomic Diagnosis: (Supraconal ☐, Conal ☐, Cauda Equina ☐)

General Autonomic Function

System/Organ	Findings	Abnormal conditions	Check mark
Autonomic control of the heart	Normal		
	Abnormal	Bradycardia	
		Tachycardia	
		Other dysrhythmias	
	Unknown		
	Unable to assess		
Autonomic control of blood pressure	Normal		
	Abnormal	Resting systolic blood pressure below 90 mmHg	
		Orthostatic hypotension	
		Autonomic dysreflexia	
	Unknown		
	Unable to assess		
Autonomic control of sweating	Normal		
	Abnormal	Hyperhydrosis above lesion	
		Hyperhydrosis below lesion	
		Hypohydrosis below lesion	
	Unknown		
	Unable to assess		
Temperature regulation	Normal		
	Abnormal	Hyperthermia	
		Hypothermia	
	Unknown		
	Unable to assess		
Autonomic and Somatic Control of Broncho-pulmonary System	Normal		
	Abnormal	Unable to voluntarily breathe requiring full ventilatory support	
		Impaired voluntary breathing requiring partial vent support	
		Voluntary respiration impaired does not require vent support	
	Unknown		

Lower Urinary Tract, Bowel and Sexual Function

System/Organ	Score
Lower Urinary Tract	
Awareness of the need to empty the bladder	
Ability to prevent leakage (continence)	
Bladder emptying method _____ (specify)	
Bowel	
Sensation of need for a bowel movement	
Ability to Prevent Stool Leakage (Continence)	
Voluntary sphincter contraction	
Sexual Function	
Genital arousal (erection or lubrication) Psychogenic	
Reflex	
Orgasm	
Ejaculation (male only)	
Sensation of Menses (female only)	

2 = Normal function, 1=Reduced or Altered Neurological Function
0=Complete loss of control NT=Unable to assess due to preexisting or concomitant problems

Urodynamic Evaluation

System/Organ	Findings	Check mark
Sensation during filling	Normal	
	Increased	
	Reduced	
	Absent	
	Non-specific	
Detrusor Activity	Normal	
	Overactive	
	Underactive	
	Acontractile	
Sphincter	Normal urethral closure mechanism	
	Normal urethral function during voiding	
	Incompetent	
	Detrusor sphincter dyssynergia	
	Non-relaxing sphincter	

Date of Injury_____   Date of Assessment_____   Examiner_____

This form may be freely copied and reproduced but not modified (Sp Cord, 2009, 47, 36-43)
This assessment should use the terminology found in the International SCI Data Set
(ASIA and ISCoS - http://www.asia-spinalinjury.org/bulletinBoard/dataset.php)

Fig 3.2-2 American Spinal Injury Association: Assessment of autonomic function.

Walking

....

Ambulation is an important functional outcome measure as it dramatically impacts patient independence and quality of life [19]. Length and speed of ambulation provides an easily quantifiable measure of function, allowing for postoperative or posttraumatic progress to be tracked in a quick and objective manner. Classical neurological exam improvements (strength and sensation) often do not translate into gait improvements, so it is important to specifically assess ability in ambulation [20].

Numerous scales have been developed to assess ambulation. These tests can be categorized into velocity dependent measures and categorical measures [21]. Velocity based measures can be further subdivided into fixed distance measures and fixed time measures. Fixed distance tests include the 10-meter walk test (10MWT) [22], the 30-meter walk test (30MWT) [23], the 50-foot walk test (50FWT) [24], and the timed up and go test (TUG) [25]. Fixed time tests include the 6-minute walk test (6MWT) [22] and the 10-second step test (10SST) [26]. Though different in distances and descriptions, these tests have been found to be strongly correlated to one another.

The categorical measures are more variable. The walking index for spinal injury (WISC-II) scale is a commonly used categorical measure based on the aids required for ambulation [27]. Points are lost as more assistance is required to complete a set distance. This scale was initially developed for spinal cord injury and has been well validated. A measurement tool called the spinal cord injury functional ambulation inventory (SCI-FAI) incorporates gait analysis, assistive device use, and both a mobility score and a distance measurement [28]. Ambulation is a component of some of the general functional assessments including the functional independence measure (FIM), spinal cord independence measure (SCIM), and the Rivermead mobility index (RMI). These functional tests are discussed in a separate portion of this chapter.

Significant disagreement exists regarding which tests should be used. The National Institute on Disability and Rehabilitation Research conference of SCI outcomes attempted to develop a consensus on walking scales [29]. Based purely on the opinions of those present, the 10MWT and the WISC-II are preferred. Although many of these scales are similar, knowledge of the details allows better understanding of outcome data and better selection for clinical use.

Composite and functional scores

The ASIA/IMSOP impairment scale is a multifaceted classification system of spinal cord injury created by the American Spinal Injury Association (ASIA) in collaboration with the International Medical Society of Paraplegia (IMSOP) and with the input of representatives from several subspecialties involved in spinal cord injury patient care. The ASIA/IMSOP grading system is now accepted as the standard grading system of spinal cord injury. It is a modified and standardized revision of the 1970's Frankel Classification system. It has strong prognostic value and heightened interobserver reliability. This A–E graded system classifies spinal cord injuries based on the degree of motor and sensory loss. It defines both extent of injury (complete, incomplete, or normal) as well as clinical syndrome (central cord, Brown-Sequard, anterior cord, conus medullaris, and cauda equina). ASIA A, or a complete spinal cord injury, is unambigiously defined as "no motor or sensory function preserved in the sacral segments S4–S5". This is an improvement over prior classification systems since it allows for an objective assessment and definitive interpretation of whether or not a patient has a complete spine injury.

While the ASIA scale remains the dominant grading system of spinal cord injury, there are also notable scales of functional outcome. The FIM includes motor and cognitive tasks and is targeted towards function and independence. The FIM is supported by a large body of data confirming its reliability and validity [30]. The SCIM is similar to the FIM, but instead of focusing on the burden of care, it addresses functional achievement and its importance to the patient [31, 32]. While ambulating with a walker may require a larger burden of care than using a wheelchair, it may also be of greater functional importance to the patient. An alternative grading system is the Barthel index and the Fugl-Meyer assessment. The Barthel index was originally intended for patients with neuromuscular disorders and is based on activities of daily living [33]. The Fugl-Meyer assessment quantifies motor recovery, balance, sensation, range of motion, and pain [34]. It is used as a whole or in part and is tailored more towards research than day-to-day clinical examination.

Summary

In this chapter, we have described commonly used scales of spinal function and discussed the reliability, correlations, strengths, and limitations of these tests. Scoring systems provide a quantifiable means of assessing prognosis, progress, and recovery, and allows for consistency between examiners and examinations. An understanding of the intended use and supporting literature of a scoring system will allow for a better tailored and more reliable choice of scale in both research and clinical practice. Based on a review of the literature, the authors would advise that the ASIA scoring system be used routinely as a new standard and not solely in the spine trauma setting, in order to document the neurological examination in patients with spinal cord and cauda equina pathology.

References

1. **Medical Research Council** (1943) *Aids to the Investigation of Peripheral Nerve Injuries.* Her Majesty's Stationery Office: London.
2. **Hislop HJ, Montgomery J** (2002) *Daniels and Worthingham's Muscle Testing: Techniques of Manual Examination.* Saunders: Philadelphia.
3. **van der Ploeg RJ, Oosterhuis HJ, Reuvekamp J** (1984) Measuring muscle strength. *J Neurol*; 231:200–203.
4. **Resnick JS, Mammel M, Mundale MO, et al** (1981) Muscular strength as an index of response to therapy in childhood dermatomyositis. *Arch Phys Med Rehabil*; 62:12–19.
5. **MacAvoy MC, Green DP** (2007) Critical reappraisal of Medical Research Council muscle testing for elbow flexion. *J Hand Surg Am*; 32:149–153.
6. **Kalsi-Ryan S, Beaton D, Curt A, et al** (2008) Quantification, sensitivity, and reliability for the sensory module of the Graded and Redefined Assessment of Sensibility Strength and Prehension (GRASSP) hand measure. In *Spinal Cord: Function, Repair, and Rehabilitation after Injury:* Montreal.
7. **Priebe MM, Waring WP** (1991) The interobserver reliability of the revised American Spinal Injury Association standards for neurological classification of spinal injury patients. *Am J Phys Med Rehabil*; 70:268–270.
8. **Krassioukov A, Wolfe DL, Hsieh JT, et al** (1999) Quantitative sensory testing in patients with incomplete spinal cord injury. *Arch Phys Med Rehabil*; 80:1258–1263.
9. **Hallett M** (1993) NINDS myotatic reflex scale. *Neurology*; 43:2723.
10. **Litvan I, Mangone CA, Werden W, et al** (1996) Reliability of the NINDS Myotatic Reflex Scale. *Neurology*; 47:969–972.
11. **Manschot S, van Passel L, Buskens E, et al** (1998) Mayo and NINDS scales for assessment of tendon reflexes: between observer agreement and implications for communication. *J Neurol Neurosurg Psychiatry*; 64:253–255.
12. **Bastron JA, Bickford RG, Brown JR, et al** (1956) *Clinical Examinations in Neurology.* Saunders: Philadelphia.
13. **Allison SC, Abraham LD, Petersen CL** (1996) Reliability of the Modified Ashworth Scale in the assessment of plantarflexor muscle spasticity in patients with traumatic brain injury. *Int J Rehabil Res*; 19:67–78.
14. **Bohannon RW, Smith MB** (1987) Interrater reliability of a modified Ashworth scale of muscle spasticity. *Phys Ther*; 67:206–207.
15. **Sloan RL, Sinclair E, Thompson J, et al** (1992) Inter-rater reliability of the modified Ashworth Scale for spasticity in hemiplegic patients. *Int J Rehabil Res*; 15:158–161.
16. **Biering-Sorensen F, Nielsen JB, Klinge K** (2006) Spasticity-assessment: a review. *Spinal Cord*; 44:708–722.
17. **Cook C, Roman M, Stewart KM, et al** (2009) Reliability and diagnostic accuracy of clinical special tests for myelopathy in patients seen for cervical dysfunction. *J Orthop Sports Phys Ther*; 39:172–178.
18. **Alexander MS, Biering-Sorensen F, Bodner D, et al** (2009) International standards to document remaining autonomic function after spinal cord injury. *Spinal Cord*; 47:36–43.
19. **Westgren N, Levi R** (1998) Quality of life and traumatic spinal cord injury. *Arch Phys Med Rehabil*; 79:1433–1439.
20. **Middleton JW, Harvey LA, Batty J, et al** (2006) Five additional mobility and locomotor items to improve responsiveness of the FIM in wheelchair-dependent individuals with spinal cord injury. *Spinal Cord*; 44:495–504.
21. **Lam T, Noonan VK, Eng JJ** (2008) A systematic review of functional ambulation outcome measures in spinal cord injury. *Spinal Cord*; 46:246–254.
22. **van Hedel HJ, Wirz M, Curt A** (2006) Improving walking assessment in subjects with an incomplete spinal cord injury: responsiveness. *Spinal Cord*; 44:352–356.
23. **Singh A, Crockard HA** (1999) Quantitative assessment of cervical spondylotic myelopathy by a simple walking test. *Lancet*; 354:370–373.
24. **Butland RJ, Pang J, Gross ER, et al** (1982) Two-, six-, and 12-minute walking tests in respiratory disease. *Br Med J (Clin Res Ed)*; 284:1607–1608.
25. **van Hedel HJ, Wirz M, Dietz V** (2005) Assessing walking ability in subjects with spinal cord injury: validity and reliability of 3 walking tests. *Arch Phys Med Rehabil*; 86:190–196.
26. **Yukawa Y, Kato F, Ito K, et al** (2009) "Ten second step test" as a new quantifiable parameter of cervical myelopathy. *Spine (Phila Pa 1976)*; 34:82–86.
27. **Morganti B, Scivoletto G, Ditunno P, et al** (2005) Walking index for spinal cord injury (WISCI): criterion validation. *Spinal Cord*; 43:27–33.
28. **Field-Fote EC, Fluet GG, Schafer SD, et al** (2001) The Spinal Cord Injury Functional Ambulation Inventory (SCI-FAI). *J Rehabil Med*; 33:177–181.
29. **Jackson AB, Carnel CT, Ditunno JF, et al** (2008) Outcome measures for gait and ambulation in the spinal cord injury population. *J Spinal Cord Med*; 31:487–499.
30. **Dodds TA, Martin DP, Stolov WC, et al** (1993) A validation of the functional independence measurement and its performance among rehabilitation inpatients. *Arch Phys Med Rehabil*; 74:531–536.
31. **Catz A, Itzkovich M, Agranov E, et al** (1997) SCIM—spinal cord independence measure: a new disability scale for patients with spinal cord lesions. *Spinal Cord*; 35:850–856.
32. **Catz A, Itzkovich M, Agranov E, et al** (2001) The spinal cord independence measure (SCIM): sensitivity to functional changes in subgroups of spinal cord lesion patients. *Spinal Cord*; 39:97–100.
33. **Mahoney FI, Barthel DW** (1965) Functional Evaluation: the Barthel Index. *Md State Med J*; 14:61–65.
34. **Duncan PW, Propst M, Nelson SG** (1983) Reliability of the Fugl-Meyer assessment of sensorimotor recovery following cerebrovascular accident. *Phys Ther*; 63:1606–1610.

3.2.1   Motor

1   Medical Research Council grading system

Description
A 5-point ordinal scale ranging from 0 to 5:
- Grade 0—No contraction
- Grade 1—Perceptible contraction in muscle, but no movement
- Grade 2—Gravity-eliminated range of motion
- Grade 3—Against gravity range of motion
- Grade 4—Motion against resistance
- Grade 5—Normal strength

Interpretation
The higher the number, the better the strength.

Clinical relevance
Detects functional weakness and assists in the identification of the neurological lesion based on specific muscle group weakness.

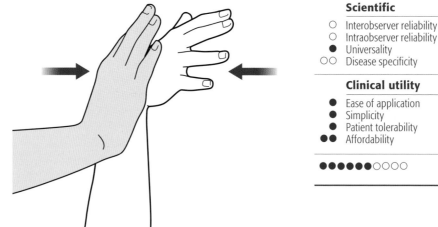

Fig 3.2.1-1

SCORING   *10 total points*

Scientific   *5 points*
- ○ Interobserver reliability
- ○ Intraobserver reliability
- ● Universality
- ○○ Disease specificity

Clinical utility   *5 points*
- ● Ease of application
- ● Simplicity
- ● Patient tolerability
- ●● Affordability

●●●●●●○○○○   **6**

Reliability

Population tested in	Interobserver reliability	Intraobserver reliability
Not tested		

2   Hand-held dynamometer

Description
A portable and objective tool to measure grip strength. Can be used bilaterally to compare relative strength differences.

Interpretation
The greater the value, the greater the strength.

Clinical relevance
Assessment of grip strength.

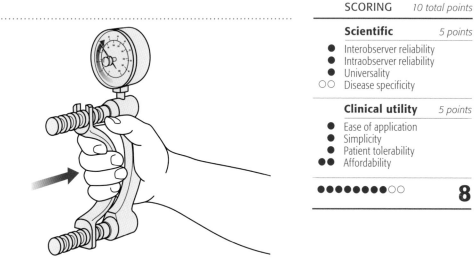

Fig 3.2.1-2

SCORING   *10 total points*

Scientific   *5 points*
- ● Interobserver reliability
- ● Intraobserver reliability
- ● Universality
- ○○ Disease specificity

Clinical utility   *5 points*
- ● Ease of application
- ● Simplicity
- ● Patient tolerability
- ●● Affordability

●●●●●●●●○○   **8**

Reliability

Population tested in	Interobserver reliability	Intraobserver reliability
Spinal cord injury patients (N=29) measured twice by four observers: two experienced physical therapists and two student physical therapists [1]	+	+
Children with spina bifida (N=20) measured by three observers: two experienced physical therapists and one student physical therapist [2]	+	NA
Spinal cord injury patients (N=25) measured twice on the same day by one observer [3]	NA	+

References:
1. **Larson CA, Tezak WD, Malley MS, et al** (2010) Assessment of postural muscle strength in sitting: reliability of measures obtained with hand-held dynamometry in individuals with spinal cord injury. *J Neurol Phys Ther;* 34:24–31.
2. **Mahony K, Hunt A, Daley D, et al** (2009) Inter-tester reliability and precision of manual muscle testing and hand-held dynamometry in lower limb muscles of children with spina bifida. *Phys Occup Ther Pediatr;* 29:44–59.
3. **May LA, Burnham RS, Steadward RD** (1997) Assessment of isokinetic and hand-held dynamometer measures of shoulder rotator strength among individuals with spinal cord injury. *Arch Phys Med Rehabil;* 78:251–255.

3   Wolf motor function test (WMF) [1]

Description
Laboratory-based measurement to
assess upper extremity motor function.
Contains 15 function-based tasks and
two strength-based tasks.
Maximum time allowed to complete
task is 120 seconds.
Scored on a 5-point ordinal scale
ranging from 0 to 5.

Interpretation
The higher the score, the greater the
function.

Clinical relevance
Allows the functional assessment of
strength and dexterity of the upper
extremities.

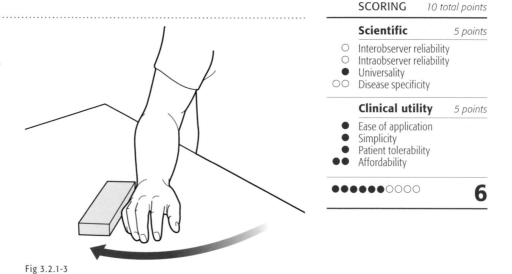

Fig 3.2.1-3

SCORING   *10 total points*

Scientific   *5 points*
○ Interobserver reliability
○ Intraobserver reliability
● Universality
○○ Disease specificity

Clinical utility   *5 points*
● Ease of application
● Simplicity
● Patient tolerability
●● Affordability

●●●●●●○○○○   **6**

Reliability

Population tested in	Interobserver reliability	Intraobserver reliability
Not tested		

References:
1. Wolf SL, Lecraw DE, Barton LA, et al (1989) Forced use of hemiplegic upper extremities to reverse the effect of learned nonuse among chronic stroke and head-injured patients. *Exp Neurol;* 104:125–132.

4   Jebsen-Taylor hand function test (JTHF) [1]

Description
Patient-completed, staff-timed measure involving seven major hand activities:
- Feeding
- Writing
- Turning pages
- Stacking checkers
- Picking up small objects
- Picking up large light objects
- Picking up large heavy objects

Both hands are tested to assess the effectiveness of specific treatments.

Interpretation
The greater the time taken, the greater the disability.

Clinical relevance
Allows the functional assessment of strength and dexterity of the upper extremities.

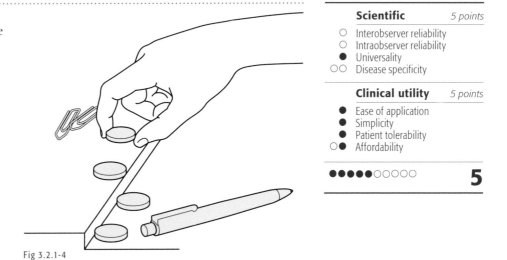

Fig 3.2.1-4

SCORING   *10 total points*

Scientific   *5 points*
- ○ Interobserver reliability
- ○ Intraobserver reliability
- ● Universality
- ○○ Disease specificity

Clinical utility   *5 points*
- ● Ease of application
- ● Simplicity
- ● Patient tolerability
- ○● Affordability

●●●●●○○○○○   **5**

Reliability

Population tested in	Interobserver reliability	Intraobserver reliability
Not tested		

References:
1. Jebsen RH, Taylor N, Trieschmann RB, et al (1969) An objective and standardized test of hand function. *Arch Phys Med Rehabil;* 50:311–319.

5   9-hole peg test

Description
A simple, timed test of fine motor coordination. The test involves the subject placing nine dowels in nine holes. Subjects are scored on the amount of time it takes to place and remove all nine pegs.

Interpretation
The greater the time taken, the greater the disability.

Clinical relevance
Allows the functional assessment of the dexterity of the upper extremities.

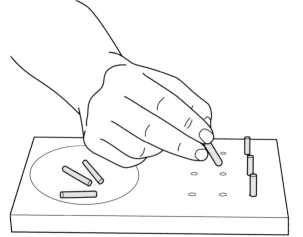

Fig 3.2.1-5

Reliability

Population tested in	Interobserver reliability	Intraobserver reliability
Not tested		

SCORING   *10 total points*

Scientific   *5 points*
- ○ Interobserver reliability
- ○ Intraobserver reliability
- ● Universality
- ○○ Disease specificity

Clinical utility   *5 points*
- ● Ease of application
- ● Simplicity
- ● Patient tolerability
- ○● Affordability

●●●●●○○○○○   **5**

6 Graded and redefined assessment of strength, sensibility and prehension (GRASSP) [1]

Description
A battery of tests quantifying upper extremity function within the following domains:
- Strength: manual muscle testing of ten muscles of the upper limb
- Sensation: Semmes-Weinstein monofilament testing
- Prehension: qualitative description of relevant finger/hand positioning for grasping and grasping test with six activities of daily life

Interpretation
Scoring and interpretation of GRASSP has been completed with pending dissemination via four manuscripts.

Clinical relevance
Allows the functional assessment of strength, dexterity, and sensation of the upper extremities, particularly after a spinal cord injury.

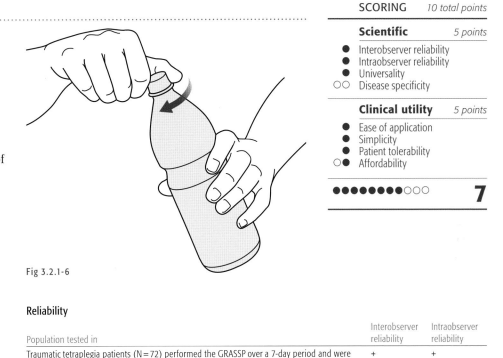

Fig 3.2.1-6

SCORING *10 total points*

Scientific *5 points*
- ● Interobserver reliability
- ● Intraobserver reliability
- ● Universality
- ○○ Disease specificity

Clinical utility *5 points*
- ● Ease of application
- ● Simplicity
- ● Patient tolerability
- ○● Affordability

●●●●●●●○○○ **7**

Reliability

Population tested in	Interobserver reliability	Intraobserver reliability
Traumatic tetraplegia patients (N = 72) performed the GRASSP over a 7-day period and were assessed by two observers: a physical therapist and an occupational therapist [2]	+	+

References:
1. **Kalsi-Ryan S, Curt A, Fehlings M, et al** (2009) Assessment of the hand tetraplegia using the Graded Redefined Assessment of Strength Sensibility and Prehension (GRASSP): Impairment versus function. *SCI Rehab;* 14:34–46.
2. **Kalsi-Ryan S, Beaton D, Curt A, et al** (2011) The Graded Redefined Assessment of Strength Sensibility and Prehension (GRASSP)—Reliability and Validity. *J Neurotrauma.*

3.2.2   Sensory

1   American Spinal Injury Association (ASIA) impairment scale—sensory

Description
Incorporates a summed score for all dermatomes using light touch and pin prick. Scored on a 0 (no sensation), 1 (reduced sensation), 2 (sensation).

Interpretation
The lower the score, the greater the sensory deficit.

Clinical relevance
Allows the grading of the magnitude of the sensory deficit.

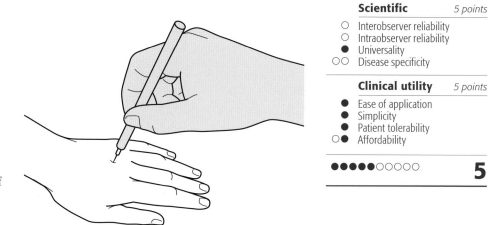

Fig 3.2.2-1

SCORING	10 total points

Scientific	5 points
○ Interobserver reliability	
○ Intraobserver reliability	
● Universality	
○○ Disease specificity	

Clinical utility	5 points
● Ease of application	
● Simplicity	
● Patient tolerability	
○● Affordability	

●●●●●○○○○○   **5**

Reliability

Population tested in	Interobserver reliability	Intraobserver reliability
Not tested		

2   Quantitative sensory testing (QST)

Description
Assess and quantify sensory function
in patients with neurological
symptoms.

Measures the detection threshold of
accurately calibrated sensory stimuli:
- Vibrations
- Thermal
- Pain

Interpretation
The lower the detection threshold, the
greater the neurological injury.

Clinical relevance
Elevated and abnormal QST
measurements may help in diagnosing
and assessing the severity of nerve
damage.

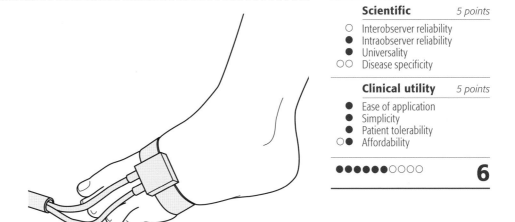

Fig 3.2.2-2

SCORING   *10 total points*

Scientific   *5 points*
- ○ Interobserver reliability
- ● Intraobserver reliability
- ● Universality
- ○○ Disease specificity

Clinical utility   *5 points*
- ● Ease of application
- ● Simplicity
- ● Patient tolerability
- ○● Affordability

●●●●●●○○○○   **6**

Reliability

Population tested in	Interobserver reliability	Intraobserver reliability
Spinal cord injury patients (N=10) were measured for mechanical, vibration, and pain thresholds twice 3 weeks apart [1]	NA	+
Spinal cord injury patients (N=21) and able-bodied controls (N=14) were measured for mechanical, vibration, and pain thresholds twice on 2 different days [2]	NA	+

References:
1. Felix ER, Widerstrom-Noga EG (2009) Reliability and validity of quantitative sensory testing in persons with spinal cord injury and neuropathic pain. *J Rehabil Res Dev;* 46:69–83.
2. Krassioukov A, Wolfe DL, Hsieh JT, et al (1999) Quantitative sensory testing in patients with incomplete spinal cord injury. *Arch Phys Med Rehabil;* 80:1258–1263.

3.2.3   Tone and reflexes

---

1   National Institute of Neurological Disorders and Stroke (NINDS) myotactic reflex scale

Description
A measurement of deep tendon reflexes. A 5-point scale that ranges from no reflex (0) to more than normal without clonus (4+).

Interpretation
The greater the score, the higher the likelihood of an upper motor neuron injury.

Clinical relevance
Allows a grading of the severity of the neurological injury.

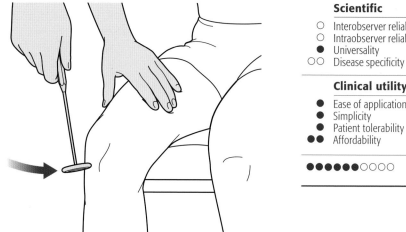

Fig 3.2.3-1

SCORING   *10 total points*

Scientific   *5 points*
○ Interobserver reliability
○ Intraobserver reliability
● Universality
○○ Disease specificity

Clinical utility   *5 points*
● Ease of application
● Simplicity
● Patient tolerability
●● Affordability

●●●●●●○○○○   **6**

Reliability

Population tested in	Interobserver reliability	Intraobserver reliability
Not tested		

2 Ashworth scale [1]

Description
Scorings system for spasticity. Measures tone and rigidity in a 5-point ordinal scale ranging from no increase in tone to rigid in flexion or extension.

Interpretation
The higher the score, the higher the spasticity.

Clinical relevance
Allows one to grade the level of spasticity.

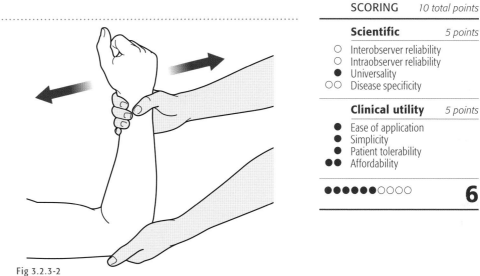

Fig 3.2.3-2

SCORING	10 total points

Scientific	5 points
○ Interobserver reliability	
○ Intraobserver reliability	
● Universality	
○○ Disease specificity	

Clinical utility	5 points
● Ease of application	
● Simplicity	
● Patient tolerability	
●● Affordability	

●●●●●●○○○○ **6**

Reliability

Population tested in	Interobserver reliability	Intraobserver reliability
Spinal cord injury patients (N = 30) were evaluated by six observers [2]	-	NA
Chronic spinal cord injury patients (N = 20) were evaluated by two blinded observers at the same time of day, weekly for 5 weeks [3]*	-	-
Spinal cord injury patients (N = 30) were evaluated by a doctor and a physical therapist [4]*	-	NA

* Modified Ashworth scale tested for reliability

References:
1. **Ashworth B** (1964) Preliminary Trial of Carisoprodol in Multiple Sclerosis. *Practitioner;* 192:540–542.
2. **Tederko P, Krasuski M, Czech J, et al** (2007) Reliability of clinical spasticity measurements in patients with cervical spinal cord injury. *Ortop Traumatol Rehabil;* 9:467–483.
3. **Craven BC, Morris AR** (2010) Modified Ashworth scale reliability for measurement of lower extremity spasticity among patients with SCI. *Spinal Cord;* 48:207–213.
4. **Haas BM, Bergstrom E, Jamous A, et al** (1996) The inter rater reliability of the original and of the modified Ashworth scale for the assessment of spasticity in patients with spinal cord injury. *Spinal Cord;* 34:560–564.

3.2.4   Autonomic

1   ASIA impairment scale—autonomic

Description
Muscle strength grading:
- 0—Total paralysis
- 1—Palpable or visible contraction
- 2—Active movement, full range of motion, gravity eliminated
- 3—Active movement, full range of motion, against gravity
- 4—Active movement, full range of motion, against gravity and provides some resistance
- 5—Active movement, full range of motion, against gravity and provides normal resistance

Interpretation
The lower the score, the greater the disability.

Clinical relevance
Grades the severity of autonomic dysfunction as a result of spinal cord injury.

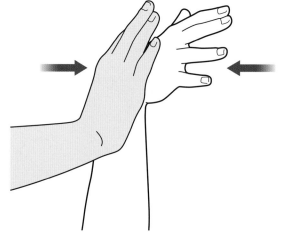

Fig 3.2.4-1

Reliability

Population tested in	Interobserver reliability	Intraobserver reliability
Not tested		

SCORING   *10 total points*

Scientific   *5 points*
- ○ Interobserver reliability
- ○ Intraobserver reliability
- ● Universality
- ○○ Disease specificity

Clinical utility   *5 points*
- ● Ease of application
- ● Simplicity
- ● Patient tolerability
- ○● Affordability

●●●●●○○○○○   **5**

3.2.5 Walking

1   10-meter walk test (10MWT) [1]

Description
Measure of time in seconds to walk 10 meters.

Interpretation
The greater the time, the greater the disability.

Clinical relevance
Provides a general assessment of ambulatory function in both neurological and orthopaedic pathologies.

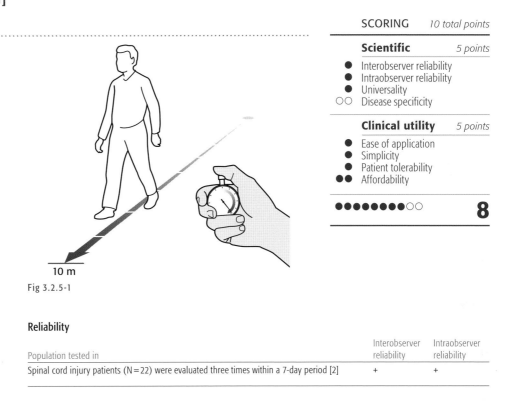

10 m

Fig 3.2.5-1

SCORING	10 total points

Scientific	5 points
● Interobserver reliability	
● Intraobserver reliability	
● Universality	
○○ Disease specificity	

Clinical utility	5 points
● Ease of application	
● Simplicity	
● Patient tolerability	
●● Affordability	

●●●●●●●●○○   **8**

Reliability

Population tested in	Interobserver reliability	Intraobserver reliability
Spinal cord injury patients (N = 22) were evaluated three times within a 7-day period [2]	+	+

References:
1. van Hedel HJ, Wirz M, Curt A (2006) Improving walking assessment in subjects with an incomplete spinal cord injury: responsiveness. *Spinal Cord;* 44:352–356.
2. van Hedel HJ, Wirz M, Dietz V (2005) Assessing walking ability in subjects with spinal cord injury: validity and reliability of 3 walking tests. *Arch Phys Med Rehabil;* 86:190–196.

2   30-meter walk test (30MWT) [1]

Description
Measure of time in seconds to walk
30 meters.

Interpretation
The greater the time, the greater the
disability.

Clinical relevance
Provides a general assessment of
ambulatory function.

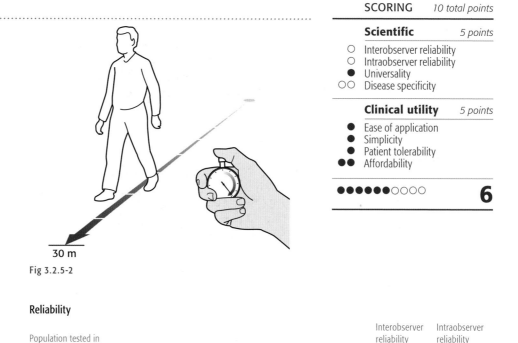

30 m

Fig 3.2.5-2

Reliability

Population tested in	Interobserver reliability	Intraobserver reliability
Not tested		

References:
1. **Singh A, Crockard HA** (1999) Quantitative assessment of cervical spondylotic myelopathy by a simple walking test. *Lancet;* 354:370–373.

3   50-foot walk test (50FWT) [1]

Description
Measure of time in seconds to walk 50 feet.

Interpretation
The greater the time, the greater the disability.

Clinical relevance
Provides a general assessment of ambulatory function.

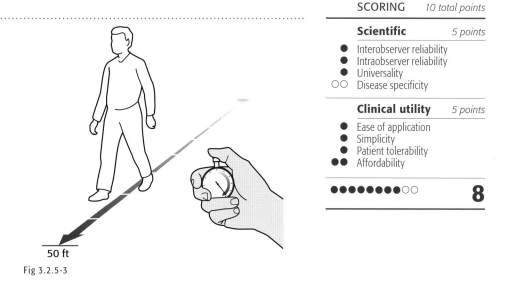

50 ft

Fig 3.2.5-3

SCORING   *10 total points*

Scientific   *5 points*
● Interobserver reliability
● Intraobserver reliability
● Universality
○○ Disease specificity

Clinical utility   *5 points*
● Ease of application
● Simplicity
● Patient tolerability
●● Affordability

●●●●●●●●○○   **8**

Reliability

Population tested in	Interobserver reliability	Intraobserver reliability
Low back pain patients (N = 44) and healthy pain-free controls (N = 48) were assessed twice 2 weeks apart by two physical therapists [2]	+	+

References:
1. Butland RJ, Pang J, Gross ER, et al (1982) Two-, six-, and 12-minute walking tests in respiratory disease. *Br Med J (Clin Res Ed);* 284:1607–1608.
2. Simmonds MJ, Olson SL, Jones S, et al (1998) Psychometric characteristics and clinical usefulness of physical performance tests in patients with low back pain. *Spine (Phila Pa 1976);* 23:2412–2421.

4   Timed up and go test (TUG) [1]

Description
Measure of time in seconds to stand up from a chair, walk 3 meters, return to the chair, and sit down.

Interpretation
Total score is the time in seconds needed to complete the task. The greater the time, the greater the disability.

Clinical relevance
Provides a general assessment of basic transfer and ambulatory function.

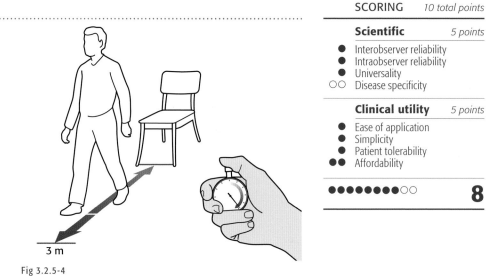

3 m

Fig 3.2.5-4

SCORING   *10 total points*

Scientific   *5 points*
● Interobserver reliability
● Intraobserver reliability
● Universality
○○ Disease specificity

Clinical utility   *5 points*
● Ease of application
● Simplicity
● Patient tolerability
●● Affordability

●●●●●●●●○○   **8**

Reliability

Population tested in	Interobserver reliability	Intraobserver reliability
Spinal cord injury patients (N=22) were evaluated three times within a 7-day period [1]	+	+
Low back pain patients (N=44) and healthy pain-free controls (N=48) were assessed twice 2 weeks apart by two physical therapists [2]	+	+

References:
1. van Hedel HJ, Wirz M, Dietz V (2005) Assessing walking ability in subjects with spinal cord injury: validity and reliability of 3 walking tests. *Arch Phys Med Rehabil;* 86:190–196.
2. Simmonds MJ, Olson SL, Jones S, et al (1998) Psychometric characteristics and clinical usefulness of physical performance tests in patients with low back pain. *Spine (Phila Pa 1976);* 23:2412–2421.

5   10-second step test (10SST)

Description
The number of steps completed in
10 seconds.

Interpretation
The fewer the steps, the greater the
disability.

Clinical relevance
Assessment of gait balance and general
ambulatory function.

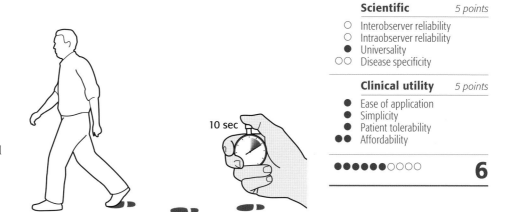

10 sec

Fig 3.2.5-5

SCORING   *10 total points*

Scientific   *5 points*
○ Interobserver reliability
○ Intraobserver reliability
● Universality
○○ Disease specificity

Clinical utility   *5 points*
● Ease of application
● Simplicity
● Patient tolerability
●● Affordability

●●●●●●○○○○   **6**

Reliability

Population tested in	Interobserver reliability	Intraobserver reliability
Not tested		

6   Walking index for spinal injury (WISC-II) [1]

Description
The following four descriptors are used when ambulating a standard distance of 10 feet:
- Ambulation devices
- Braces
- Assistance
- Patient reported comfort level

The clinician records the highest level achieved safely by the patient.

Interpretation
The total score is the highest level achieved.
- Maximum score: 20
- Minimum score: 0

The lower the score, the greater the disability.

Clinical relevance
An overall assessment of gait, balance, lower extremity function, and pain in patients with spinal cord dysfunction.

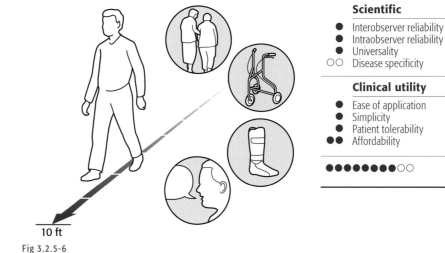

10 ft

Fig 3.2.5-6

SCORING	10 total points
Scientific	5 points

- ● Interobserver reliability
- ● Intraobserver reliability
- ● Universality
- ○○ Disease specificity

Clinical utility	5 points

- ● Ease of application
- ● Simplicity
- ● Patient tolerability
- ●● Affordability

●●●●●●●●○○   **8**

Reliability

Population tested in	Interobserver reliability	Intraobserver reliability
Spinal cord injury patients (N = 26) were tested twice on two different days by two blinded physical therapists [2]	+	+

References:
1. **Dittuno PL, Ditunno JF, Jr.** (2001) Walking index for spinal cord injury (WISCI II): scale revision. *Spinal Cord;* 39:654–656.
2. **Marino RJ, Scivoletto G, Patrick M, et al** (2010) Walking index for spinal cord injury version 2 (WISCI-II) with repeatability of the 10-m walk time: Inter- and intrarater reliabilities. *Am J Phys Med Rehabil;* 89:7–15.

7   Spinal cord injury functional ambulation inventory (SCI-FAI) [1]

Description
Nine items relating to the following
domains:
- Gait parameters (20 points)
- Assistive device use (14 points)
- Walking mobility score (5 points)

Each item scored on a scale with a
minimum score of 0 and a variable
maximum score of 1, 2, 3, 4 or 5.

A timed 2-minute walk test is added to
the walking mobility domain, but has
no bearing on the overall score.

Interpretation
Scores within each domain are
summed up to create a composite score
for that domain. These scores are not
combined for an overall composite
score.
- Maximum gait parameter score: 20
- Minimum gait parameter score: 0
- Maximum assistive device score: 14
- Minimum assistive device score: 0
- Maximum walking mobility score: 5
- Minimum walking mobility score: 0

The lower the score, the greater the
disability.

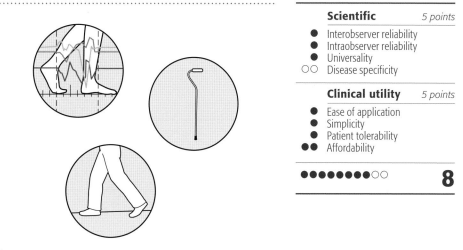

Fig 3.2.5-7

Reliability

Population tested in	Interobserver reliability	Intraobserver reliability
Spinal cord injury patients (N=22) were tested three times (once live, twice by videotape) by four physical therapists [1]	+	+

Clinical relevance
An overall assessment of gait, balance,
and lower extremity function in
patients with spinal cord dysfunction.

References:
1. Field-Fote EC, Fluet GG, Schafer SD, et al (2001) The Spinal Cord Injury Functional Ambulation Inventory (SCI-FAI).
   J Rehabil Med; 33:177–181.

3.2.6   Composite scales

---

1   ASIA/International Medical Society of Paraplegia (IMSOP)

Description

Contains five grades of impairment:

- Grade A—Complete
- Grade B—Incomplete: sensory but not motor function is preserved below the neurological level and includes the sacral segments S4/5
- Grade C—Incomplete: motor function is preserved below the neurological level, and more than half of the key muscles below the neurological level have a muscle grade less than 3 strength
- Grade D—Incomplete: motor function is preserved below the neurological level, and at least half of the key muscles below the neurological level have a muscle grade of 3 or more strength
- Grade E—Normal

Interpretation

Grades are presented in ascending order of severity.

Clinical relevance

Assess severity of spinal cord injury.

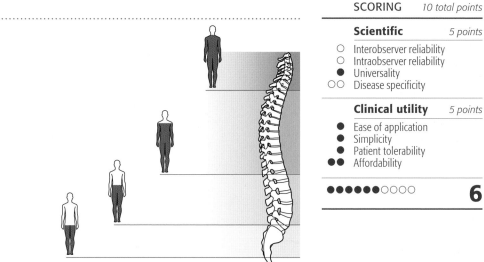

Fig 3.2.6-1

Reliability

Population tested in	Interobserver reliability	Intraobserver reliability
Not tested		

SCORING   *10 total points*

Scientific   *5 points*
- ○ Interobserver reliability
- ○ Intraobserver reliability
- ● Universality
- ○○ Disease specificity

Clinical utility   *5 points*
- ● Ease of application
- ● Simplicity
- ● Patient tolerability
- ●● Affordability

●●●●●●○○○○   **6**

2   Functional independence measure (FIM) [1]

SCORING   *10 total points*

Description
18 items relating to the following categories:
- Self-care (42 points)
- Sphincter control (14 points)
- Transfers (7 points)
- Mobility (14 points)
- Locomotion (14 points)
- Communication and cognition (35 points)

Each item scored on a 1 to 7 point scale.

Interpretation
Total score is the sum of all items.
- Maximum score: 126
- Minimum score: 18

The lower the score, the greater the disability.

Clinical relevance
A global assessment of daily physical and cognitive function often used for determining the need for additional supportive care.

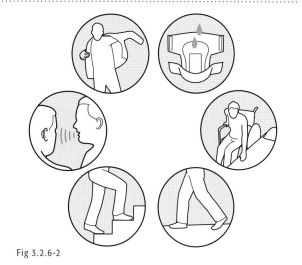

Fig 3.2.6-2

Scientific   *5 points*
- ○ Interobserver reliability
- ○ Intraobserver reliability
- ● Universality
- ○○ Disease specificity

Clinical utility   *5 points*
- ● Ease of application
- ● Simplicity
- ● Patient tolerability
- ●● Affordability

●●●●●●○○○○   **6**

Reliability

Population tested in	Interobserver reliability	Intraobserver reliability
Not tested		

References:
1. O'Toole DM, Golden AM (1991) Evaluating cancer patients for rehabilitation potential. *West J Med;* 155:384–387.

3   Spinal cord independence measure (SCIM) [1]

Description
16 items relating to the following categories:
- Self-care (20 points)
- Respiration and sphincter management (40 points)
- Mobility in room and around toilet (10 points)
- Mobility indoors and outdoors (30 points)

Each item scored on a scale with a minimum score of 0 and a variable maximum score of 2, 5, 6, 8, 10, or 15.

Interpretation
Total score is the sum of all items.
- Maximum score: 100
- Minimum score: 0

The lower the score, the greater the disability.

Clinical relevance
A global assessment of daily physical and cognitive function often used for determining the need for additional supportive care.

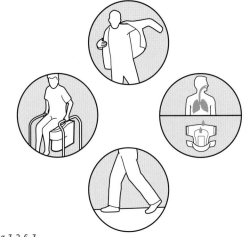

Fig 3.2.6-3

SCORING   *10 total points*

Scientific	*5 points*
● Interobserver reliability	
● Intraobserver reliability	
● Universality	
○○ Disease specificity	

Clinical utility	*5 points*
● Ease of application	
● Simplicity	
● Patient tolerability	
●● Affordability	

●●●●●●●●○○   **8**

Reliability

Population tested in	Interobserver reliability	Intraobserver reliability
Patients with spinal cord lesions (N=30) evaluated every month during admission by two observers [1]	+	+

References:
1. Catz A, Itzkovich M, Agranov E, et al (1997) SCIM—spinal cord independence measure: a new disability scale for patients with spinal cord lesions. *Spinal Cord;* 35:850–856.

4 Rivermead mobility index (RMI) [1]

Description
A measure of disability related to bodily mobility. It demonstrates the patient's ability to move her or his own body. It does not measure the effective use of a wheelchair or the mobility when aided by someone else.

Each item scored on a 0 to 1 point scale.

Interpretation
Total score is sum of all 15 questions.

The higher the score, the better the mobility.

Clinical relevance
An assessment of the patient's bed mobility, postural transfers, and walking ability. Uses a combined interview and observation format.

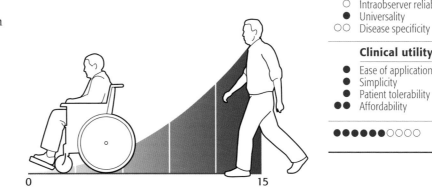

0   15

Fig 3.2.6-4

Reliability

Population tested in	Interobserver reliability	Intraobserver reliability
Not tested		

SCORING *10 total points*

Scientific *5 points*
○ Interobserver reliability
○ Intraobserver reliability
● Universality
○○ Disease specificity

Clinical utility *5 points*
● Ease of application
● Simplicity
● Patient tolerability
●● Affordability

●●●●●●○○○○ **6**

References:
1. **Collen FM, Wade DT, Robb GF, et al** (1991) The Rivermead Mobility Index: a further development of the Rivermead Motor Assessment. *Int Disabil Stud;* 13:50–54.

5   Barthel index [1]

Description
Ten items relating to the following categories:
- Self-care (30 points)
- Walking (25 points)
- Transfer (15 points)
- Controlling bowels and bladder (20 points)
- Feeding (10 points)

Each item scored a scale with a minimum score of 0 and a variable maximum score of 5, 10 or 15.

Interpretation
Total score is the sum of all items.
- Maximum score: 100
- Minimum score: 0

The lower the score, the greater the disability.

Clinical relevance
A global assessment of daily physical and cognitive function often used for determining the need for additional supportive care.

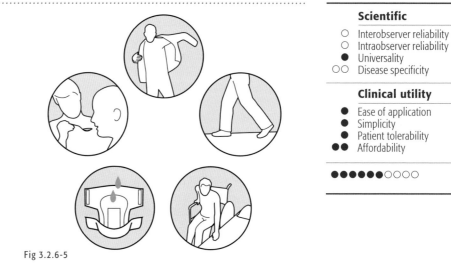

Fig 3.2.6-5

Reliability

Population tested in	Interobserver reliability	Intraobserver reliability
Not tested		

SCORING	10 total points

Scientific	5 points

- ○ Interobserver reliability
- ○ Intraobserver reliability
- ● Universality
- ○○ Disease specificity

Clinical utility	5 points

- ● Ease of application
- ● Simplicity
- ● Patient tolerability
- ●● Affordability

●●●●●●○○○○   **6**

References:
1. Mahoney FI, Barthel DW (1965) Functional Evaluation: the Barthel Index. *Md State Med J;* 14:61–65.

6   Fugl-Meyer assessment [1]

Description
A stroke-specific, performance-based impairment index. It is designed to assess motor functioning, balance, sensation, and joint functioning in patients with post-stroke hemiplegia.

Consists of 155 items, with each item rated on a 3-point ordinal scale, 2 points for the detail being performed completely, 1 point for the detail being partially completed, and 0 points for the detail not being performed.

Interpretation
A maximum score total of 226 points—100 for motor performance, 14 for balance, 24 for sensations, and 44 for passive joint motion and joint pain.

The maximum score for the motor performance is divided into 66 points for the upper extremity and 34 for the lower extremity. Less than 50 points in the motor performance equals severe motor impairment. If scores are between 50 and 84, this equals moderate impairment. If scores are between 85 and 99, this equals slight motor impairment.

Clinical relevance
Applied clinically and in research to determine disease severity, describe motor recovery, and to plan and assess treatment.

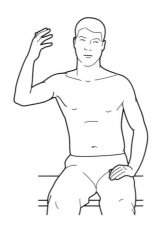 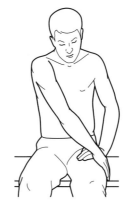

Fig 3.2.6-6

Scientific   *5 points*
○ Interobserver reliability
○ Intraobserver reliability
● Universality
○○ Disease specificity

Clinical utility   *5 points*
● Ease of application
● Simplicity
● Patient tolerability
●● Affordability

●●●●●●○○○○   **6**

Reliability

Population tested in	Interobserver reliability	Intraobserver reliability
Not tested		

References:
1. **Fugl-Meyer AR, Jaasko L, Leyman I, et al** (1975) The post-stroke hemiplegic patient. 1. a method for evaluation of physical performance. *Scand J Rehabil Med;* 7:13–31.

3   Clinical measurements
3.3   Strength measurements

3   Clinical measurements

3.3   Strength measurements

Introduction

Reasons for testing

Spine surgeons do not routinely measure spine strength, or more specifically, trunk muscle strength when assessing their patients. Simple manual testing is an option, but such tests suffer from subjectivity, lack of uniformity, and lack of quantification. More specific trunk muscle strength tests are time-consuming, often require bulky and expensive equipment, and the information gleaned is generally felt to be of limited value in routine practice. More commonly, such tests are undertaken by rehabilitation clinicians or as part of research, especially in relation to low back pain, where it is accepted that trunk muscle strength is clinically relevant [1, 2]. Some research has suggested that spine strength measurement tools may be useful in identifying risk factors, planning treatment, and measuring progress.

Types of tests

Trunk performance can be evaluated in terms of endurance and strength. Broadly speaking, endurance tests are manual examinations conducted with minimal equipment, while strength measurements are mechanized and usually computerized . These can be isometric (isotonic), isokinetic, or isodynamic (isoinertial), depending on whether the test is against a fixed resistance or through a range of movement, and whether the movement is at a fixed or variable velocity.

Endurance tests

Extension

The best-known static endurance test is the Biering-Sorensen test, which measures how many seconds a subject is able to keep the unsupported upper body in a horizontal position. The subject lies prone with the lower body supported either on a Roman chair with supports, or on a bench with straps. The subject initially has the waist flexed with the head hanging down and is asked to raise the trunk to the horizontal position with hands crossed over the chest. The test is continued until the subject can no longer maintain the horizontal position [3].

Numerous studies have shown that the test is accurate and reliable, although it is unclear whether it can discriminate between subjects with and without low back pain [4, 5]. Ito et al have described a variation of this test where the subject lies prone on the floor with a small pillow under the abdomen to reduce lumbar lordosis, and is asked to extend their trunk to keep the sternum off the floor for as long as possible [6].

A dynamic test can be performed by asking the subject to repeatedly extend and count the number of repetitions [7, 8].

Flexion

These tests evaluate flexor (abdominal) endurance. The subject lies supine and is asked to maintain about 25° upper trunk flexion (a partial crunch) or hip flexion (a partial straight leg raise). Alternately, both the upper trunk and hips can be flexed simultaneously. Time to fatigue is measured. A variation of the original Kraus-Weber fitness test, this measure is less commonly used and has been less thoroughly evaluated for accuracy and reliability. Dynamic endurance can be measured by counting the number of partial crunches that can be performed until fatigue [7].

Strength iso-tests

Isometric

The simplest strength test is isometric, where maximum force exerted against static resistance in a particular plane (eg, trunk flexion) is measured. The test can be repeated at different angles to generate a strength curve. The Tergumed system is one commonly employed isometric measurement system. Four devices consisting of fixed weight-resistance systems are used to measure flexion, extension, lateral flexion, and rotation. The subject is seated with appropriate restraints and asked to perform a maximal voluntary contraction for 6 seconds. The MedX system is a similar device. Due to the static nature of the testing, results from isometric devices are of limited value when assessing dynamic function.

Isokinetic

Isokinetic testing provides a more dynamic assessment, where force or torque is measured throughout a range of movement at various constant, preset velocities. As muscular output increases, the machine resistance increases, and acceleration is not possible. One of the best known isokinetic trunk testing machines is the Cybex, which consists of three separate machines to measure trunk extension/flexion, torso rotation, and lifting. Peak torque or force is measured at various speeds, and the software derives average power and various rations including extension/flexion and left/right rotation. Consistency of effort is derived by calculating an average points variance. Other machines that measure only trunk extension/flexion include the KIN/COM and Biodex devices. Although measurement through a range of movement more closely simulates normal function, controlling the speed of motion is somewhat unnatural, limiting the real-life relevance of the results.

Variability

Isodynamic

Isodynamic testing employs a constant force or maximum torque during movement, thereby allowing for changes in acceleration and velocity of motion in proportion to the muscular effort of the user. The Isostation B-200 device is a triaxial dynamometer that simultaneously measures lumbar movements in three axes. Although theoretically of more clinical relevance, there are practical limitations to this device and a paucity of published studies.

Computerized trunk strength tests are subject to moderate variability due to factors such as the learning effect, the amount of effort applied, and the effect of pain and emotional stress [9]. The learning effect is reflected by increased performance on subsequent testing. This can significantly influence results if not taken into consideration [10]. The learning effect is of considerable concern when monitoring treatment outcome [11]. Another confounder is the effect of deconditioning, which can mimic back pain and symptom magnification [12]. The amount of effort can depend on the willingness of the subject to exert maximum force, the subject's fear of injury, and the instructions given on how to perform the given activity [13]. Technical confounders include calibration, patient stabilization, and axis placement [14]. Other considerations are the lack of standardized protocols and normative data, and the fact that results are device specific, making comparisons between devices difficult [15].

Value

The introduction of specialized testing machines raised the prospect of adding science to spine function assessment. They would allow quantification of functional ability and allow correlation with normal values and workplace demands. Clinicians could accurately measure baseline function, assess treatment interventions, and even screen patients to assess job suitability and to identify malingerers. To date, these promises have not been fulfilled [16]. Clinically applicable differences between normal subjects and back pain patients have not been demonstrated [5, 12, 17]. Although some studies show differences in the mean measurements, the ranges are wide and overlapping with limited discrimination [10]. There is insufficient evidence that computerized muscle testing improves clinical outcome, or that the devices are superior to other exercise equipment when used to deliver treatment [18]. There are limitations in using strength testing in determining the ability to perform a physically demanding job. The test needs to be specific to the job, and even so, there are no long-term studies that confirm that a poor test result predicts an increased risk of injury. There are also legal and discrimination issues surrounding the use of such pre-employment screening. In the medicolegal sphere, strength testing has not been particularly effective as a "spinal lie detector", mainly because inconsistent results can be due to many factors other than submaximal effort [19]. Assessment of permanent impairment using strength tests has not been validated, and it is difficult to extrapolate an overall functional ability from a specific measurement of trunk muscle strength. There is a consensus that there is inadequate scientific evidence to support iso-testing [10].

As a result of these shortcomings, together with the practical considerations of time, space, and affordability associated with these devices, there has been a decline in the popularity, use, and acceptance of these systems [20].

Other strength tests

Electromyography (EMG) testing

The use of surface EMG to quantify muscle fatigue during an endurance test has been proposed as a motivation-free alternative to the usual endurance tests [21]. The EMG signal can be analyzed during a sustained contraction, and the median frequency of the EMG power spectrum and the concomitant increase of EMG amplitude can be used as indices of muscle fatigue [22, 23]. There are a number of confounding variables including the effects of pain and effort [24], and the use of EMG to measure fatigue and thus trunk strength is still in the development phase.

Cervical spine

Less work has been done in the neck when compared with the low back. Isometric testing has been reported using a modified sphygmomanometer-type dynamometer, where neck strength in flexion, extension, lateral flexion, or rotation is measured by pushing the head against an air bladder and measuring the pressure generated [25]. It has also been associated with the use of more specialized equipment [26]. Normative values have been determined for both normal and symptomatic subjects but there is little information about clinical correlation. Muscle endurance tests have been similarly evaluated [27, 28]. To date, there is insufficient evidence to support the routine use of neck strength or endurance measurement in diagnosis or treatment of neck disorders.

Summary

Strength is an expression of spinal health. In isolation, it is difficult to interpret and subject to variability. Interpretation of strength should be performed in the context of the patient's overall health. For example, two patients with identical spinal health and greatly differing appendicular musculoskeletal health, may yield completely different strength examinations. Perhaps, in the future, combining routine measures with feedback-oriented rehabilitation may further our understanding.

References

1. **Nachemson A** (1969) Physiotherapy for low back pain patients. A critical look. *Scand J Rehabil Med;* 1:85–90.

2. **McQuade KJ, Turner JA, Buchner DM** (1988) Physical fitness and chronic low back pain. An analysis of the relationships among fitness, functional limitations, and depression. *Clin Orthop Relat Res;* 233:198–204.

3. **Biering-Sorensen F** (1984) Physical measurements as risk indicators for low-back trouble over a one-year period. *Spine (Phila Pa 1976);* 9:106–119.

4. **Latimer J, Maher CG, Refshauge K, et al** (1999) The reliability and validity of the Biering-Sorensen test in asymptomatic subjects and subjects reporting current or previous nonspecific low back pain. *Spine (Phila Pa 1976);* 24:2085–2089.

5. **Keller A, Hellesnes J, Brox JI** (2001) Reliability of the isokinetic trunk extensor test, Biering-Sorensen test, and Astrand bicycle test: assessment of intraclass correlation coefficient and critical difference in patients with chronic low back pain and healthy individuals. *Spine (Phila Pa 1976);* 26:771–777.

6. **Ito T, Shirado O, Suzuki H, et al** (1996) Lumbar trunk muscle endurance testing: an inexpensive alternative to a machine for evaluation. *Arch Phys Med Rehabil;* 77:75–79.

7. **Moreland J, Finch E, Stratford P, et al** (1997) Interrater reliability of six tests of trunk muscle function and endurance. *J Orthop Sports Phys Ther;* 26:200–208.

8. **Smidt GL, Blanpied PR** (1987) Analysis of strength tests and resistive exercises commonly used for low-back disorders. *Spine;* 12:1025–1034.

9. **Mayer T, Gatchel R, Betancur J, et al** (1995) Trunk muscle endurance measurement. Isometric contrasted to isokinetic testing in normal subjects. *Spine (Phila Pa 1976);* 20:920–926.

10. **Newton M, Thow M, Somerville D, et al** (1993) Trunk strength testing with iso-machines. Part 2: Experimental evaluation of the Cybex II Back Testing System in normal subjects and patients with chronic low back pain. *Spine (Phila Pa 1976);* 18:812–824.

11. **Gruther W, Wick F, Paul B, et al** (2009) Diagnostic accuracy and reliability of muscle strength and endurance measurements in patients with chronic low back pain. *J Rehabil Med;* 41:613–619.

12. **Mandell PJ, Weitz E, Bernstein JI, et al** (1993) Isokinetic trunk strength and lifting strength measures. Differences and similarities between low-back-injured and noninjured workers. *Spine;* 18:2491–2501.

13. **Matheson L, Mooney V, Caiozzo V, et al** (1992) Effect of instructions on isokinetic trunk strength testing variability, reliability, absolute value, and predictive validity. *Spine;* 17:914–921.

14. **Stokes IA, Gookin DM, Reid S, et al** (1990) Effects of axis placement on measurement of isokinetic flexion and extension torque in the lumbar spine. *J Spinal Disord;* 3:114–118.

15. **Roussel N, Nijs J, Truijen S, et al** (2006) Reliability of the assessment of lumbar range of motion and maximal isometric strength. *Arch Phys Med Rehabil;* 87:576–582.

16. **Mooney V, Andersson GB** (1994) Trunk strength testing in patient evaluation and treatment. *Spine;* 19:2483–2485.

17. **Langrana NA, Lee CK, Alexander H, et al** (1984) Quantitative assessment of back strength using isokinetic testing. *Spine;* 9:287–290.

18. **Aetna** (2009) Clinical Policy Bulletin: Back Pain—Non Invasive Treatments.

19. **Hazard RG, Reid S, Fenwick J, et al** (1988) Isokinetic trunk and lifting strength measurements: variability as an indicator of effort. *Spine;* 13:54–57.

20. **Orri JC, Darden GF** (2008) Technical report: Reliability and validity of the iSAM 9000 isokinetic dynamometer. *J Strength Cond Res;* 22:310–317.

21. **Lariviere C, Arsenault AB, Gravel D, et al** (2002) Evaluation of measurement strategies to increase the reliability of EMG indices to assess back muscle fatigue and recovery. *J Electromyogr Kinesiol;* 12:91–102.

22. **Lariviere C, Gagnon D, Gravel D, et al** (2008) The assessment of back muscle capacity using intermittent static contractions. Part I—Validity and reliability of electromyographic indices of fatigue. *J Electromyogr Kinesiol;* 18:1006–1019.

23. **Lariviere C, Gravel D, Gagnon D, et al** (2008) The assessment of back muscle capacity using intermittent static contractions. Part II: validity and reliability of biomechanical correlates of muscle fatigue. *J Electromyogr Kinesiol;* 18:1020–1031.

24. **Pitcher MJ, Behm DG, MacKinnon SN** (2008) Reliability of electromyographic and force measures during prone isometric back extension in subjects with and without low back pain. *Appl Physiol Nutr Metab;* 33:52–60.

25. **Vernon HT, Aker P, Aramenko M, et al** (1992) Evaluation of neck muscle strength with a modified sphygmomanometer dynamometer: reliability and validity. *J Manipulative Physiol Ther;* 15:343–349.

26. **Chiu TT, Lam TH, Hedley AJ** (2002) Maximal isometric muscle strength of the cervical spine in healthy volunteers. *Clin Rehabil;* 16:772–779.

27. **Edmondston SJ, Wallumrod ME, Macleid F, et al** (2008) Reliability of isometric muscle endurance tests in subjects with postural neck pain. *J Manipulative Physiol Ther;* 31:348–54.

28. **Harris KD, Heer DM, Roy TC, et al** (2005) Reliability of a measurement of neck flexor muscle endurance. *Phys Ther;* 85:1349–1355.

3.3.1   Isometric testing

1   Tergumed system/MedX

Description
Maximum force exerted against static resistance in a particular plane (eg, trunk flexion) is measured.

Four devices consisting of fixed weight-resistance systems are used to measure flexion, extension, lateral flexion, and rotation. The subject is seated with appropriate restraints and asked to perform a maximal voluntary contraction for 6 seconds.

Interpretation
Interpretation can be based on serial testing in patients individually to track progress. Absolute standards and thresholds are difficult to define due to the paucity of scientific literature.

Clinical relevance
Due to the static nature of the testing, results from isometric devices are of limited value when assessing dynamic function.

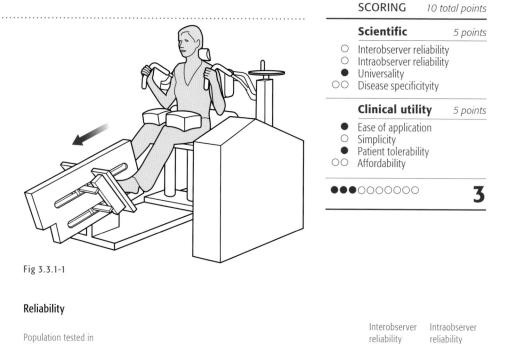

Fig 3.3.1-1

SCORING   *10 total points*

Scientific   *5 points*
- ○ Interobserver reliability
- ○ Intraobserver reliability
- ● Universality
- ○○ Disease specificityity

Clinical utility   *5 points*
- ● Ease of application
- ○ Simplicity
- ● Patient tolerability
- ○○ Affordability

●●●○○○○○○○   **3**

Reliability

Population tested in	Interobserver reliability	Intraobserver reliability
Not tested		

3.3.2   Isokinetic dynamometer

1   Biodex/Cybex/iSam 900

SCORING   *10 total points*

Description
Measures the force generated by a muscle at a constant rate of movement. Isokinetic dynamometers provide constant velocity with accommodating resistance through a joint's range of motion.

A combination of isokinetic dynamometers and computer software allows the clinician to obtain measures of muscle function related to torque, power, and endurance.

Interpretation
Measures obtained give a measure of overall muscle performance:
• Peak torque
• Power
• Endurance

Clinical relevance
Serial testing and values can track a patient's progress with overall conditioning and core strengthening.

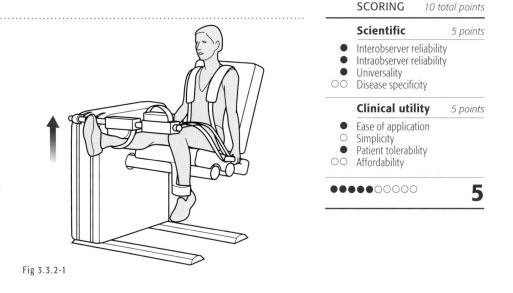

Fig 3.3.2-1

Scientific   *5 points*
● Interobserver reliability
● Intraobserver reliability
● Universality
○○ Disease specificity

Clinical utility   *5 points*
● Ease of application
○ Simplicity
● Patient tolerability
○○ Affordability

●●●●●○○○○○   **5**

Reliability

Population tested in	Interobserver reliability	Intraobserver reliability
Isometric neck muscle strength of healthy patients (N = 12) measured by Biodex isokinetic dynamometer three times one week apart by three observers: one manual therapist and two manual therapy students [1]	+	+

References:
1. Cagnie B, Cools A, De Loose V, et al (2007) Differences in isometric neck muscle strength between healthy controls and women with chronic neck pain: the use of a reliable measurement. *Arch Phys Med Rehabil;* 88:1441–1445.

3.3.3   Isodynamic testing

1   Isostation B-200 device

Description
Employs a constant force or maximum torque during movement, thereby allowing for changes in acceleration and velocity of motion in proportion to the muscular effort of the user.

The Isostation B-200 device is a triaxial dynamometer that simultaneously measures lumbar movements in three axes.

Interpretation
Interpretation can be based on serial testing in patients individually to track progress. Absolute standards and thresholds are difficult to define due to the paucity of scientific literature.

Clinical relevance
Although theoretically of more clinical relevance, there are practical limitations of this device and a paucity of published studies.

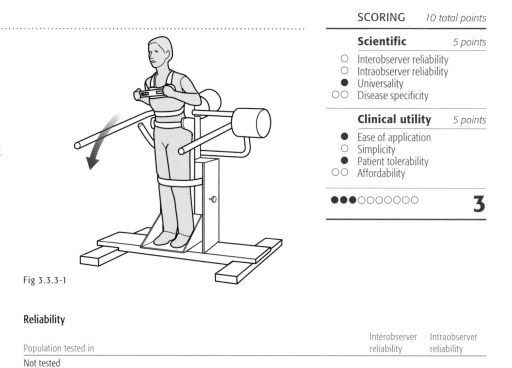

Fig 3.3.3-1

SCORING	10 total points
Scientific	5 points

○ Interobserver reliability
○ Intraobserver reliability
● Universality
○○ Disease specificity

Clinical utility	5 points

● Ease of application
○ Simplicity
● Patient tolerability
○○ Affordability

●●●○○○○○○○   **3**

Reliability

Population tested in	Interobserver reliability	Intraobserver reliability
Not tested		

3.3.4 Other strength tests

1 Biering-Sorensen back test [1]

Description
Measures how many seconds a patient is able to keep the unsupported upper body in a horizontal position. Load is equal to the weight of the upper body, with torque determined by the lever arm from the pubic symphysis to the upper body's center of gravity.

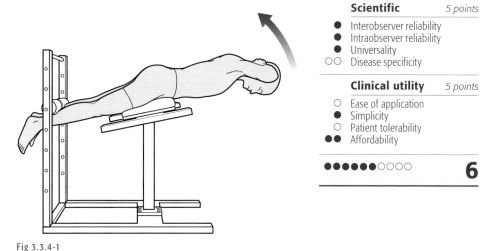

Interpretation
Test is continued until patient can no longer control horizontal posture, or until patient reaches the limit of fatigue or pain tolerance.

Fig 3.3.4-1

Clinical relevance
Serial testing and values can track a patient's progress with overall conditioning and core strengthening.

Reliability

Population tested in	Interobserver reliability	Intraobserver reliability
Biering-Sorensen back test holding position measured in varying-degree low back pain patients (N=63) twice 15 minutes apart by four observers: three manual therapists and one spine clinical practice therapist [2]	+	+
Biering-Sorensen back test measured in low back pain patients (N=31) and healthy individuals (N=31) three times 5–10 days apart by an experienced physical therapist [3]	NA	+ (LBP patients) - (healthy patients)
Biering-Sorensen back test measured in low back pain patients (N=100) and healthy individuals (N=90) by a physical therapist [4]	NA	+
Biering-Sorensen back test measured in healthy individuals (N=152) [5]	NA	-

References:
1. **Biering-Sorensen F** (1984) Physical measurements as risk indicators for low-back trouble over a one-year period. *Spine (Phila Pa 1976);* 9:106–119.
2. **Latimer J, Maher CG, Refshauge K, et al** (1999) The reliability and validity of the Biering-Sorensen test in asymptomatic subjects and subjects reporting current or previous nonspecific low back pain. *Spine (Phila Pa 1976);* 24:2085–2089; discussion 2090.
3. **Keller A, Hellesnes J, Brox JI** (2001) Reliability of the isokinetic trunk extensor test, Biering-Sorensen test, and Astrand bicycle test: assessment of intraclass correlation coefficient and critical difference in patients with chronic low back pain and healthy individuals. *Spine (Phila Pa 1976);* 26:771–777.
4. **Ito T, Shirado O, Suzuki H, et al** (1996) Lumbar trunk muscle endurance testing: an inexpensive alternative to a machine for evaluation. *Arch Phys Med Rehabil;* 77:75–79.
5. **Mayer T, Gatchel R, Betancur J, et al** (1995) Trunk muscle endurance measurement. *Isometric contrasted to isokinetic testing in normal subjects.* Spine (Phila Pa 1976); 20:920-926; discussion 926–927.

3   Clinical measurements
3.4 Body composition measurements

3   Clinical measurements

3.4   Body composition measurements

Introduction

When considering surgical management of any condition, structural body composition is of paramount importance. It is generally well known that osteoporosis and obesity pose challenges in reconstructive surgical management. In addition to the physical challenges of operating on the morbidly obese, there is greater postoperative risk for morbidity and mortality. Assessment of bone density is particularly important when considering instrumentation as mechanical failure is known to be more common in patients with low bone density. Like all other conditions, there is a spectrum of severity for bone density and obesity. This section seeks to provide a more detailed quantitative assessment of these body composition measurements.

Osteoporosis

Osteoporosis is essentially "a systemic skeletal disease characterized by low bone mass and micro-architectural deterioration of bone tissue leading to enhanced bone fragility and a consequent increase in fracture risk" [1] (**Fig 3.4-1**).

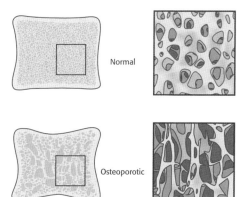

Fig 3.4-1 Normal versus osteoporotic bone.

Osteoporosis in women is defined by the World Health Organization (WHO) as a bone mineral density that is 2.5 standard deviations below peak bone mass as measured by dual energy x-ray absorptiometry (DEXA), and the term "established osteoporosis" includes the presence of a fragility fracture.

Osteoporosis is estimated to affect 200 million people worldwide, including one third of the women aged 60–70 and two thirds of the women aged over 80 [2]. The significance of this figure is that osteoporosis increases the risk of fractures, with the three most common sites being the hip, vertebral body, and wrist (**Fig 3.4-2**). Women are more commonly affected than men, with the cumulative lifetime risk of having an osteoporotic fracture being two to four times that of men [3].

The age-specific incidence of vertebral fractures may be difficult to estimate as many of the fractures are subclinical. Approximately 30% of women over the age of 50 will have one or more vertebral fractures [4]. Another study showed that the prevalence of wedge fractures in normal women to be approximately 60% [5]. With regard to the differences between the sexes, it is estimated that women will have 10 times more vertebral fractures than men [6]. The socioeconomic impact of this extremely common and widespread disease can be quite incapacitating for countries around the world (**Table 3.4-1**).

Disease	Number of sick days
Osteoporosis	701,000
Chronic obstructive pulmonary disease	891,000
Stroke	533,000
Myocardial infarction	238,000
Breast cancer	201,000

Table 3.4-1 Number of sick days and their related causes for men and women in Switzerland in 1992 [7].

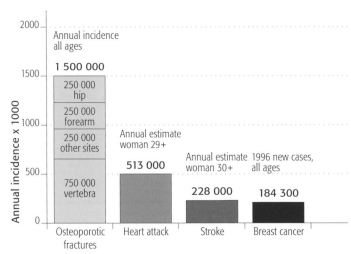

Fig 3.4-2 Osteoporotic fractures when compared to other diseases in women in the USA [8].

Measurements techniques

Bone mineral density is an important predictor of fracture risk [9, 10]. There are various techniques and methods to measure bone mineral density, using either x-ray, ultrasound, or CT-based technology. The common methods used are listed below:

- DEXA
- Ultrasound attenuation and velocity
- CT-based quantitative densitometry

While bone density values can be determined with these measurement techniques, bone properties such as brittleness may not fully correlate.

Dual energy x-ray absorptiometry (DEXA)

This test is currently regarded as the gold standard for the diagnosis of osteoporosis. It utilizes an enhanced form of x-ray technology to take images of the bone and measure the amount of bone loss. Two x-ray sources with two different beam intensities are used to measure the amount of radiation absorbed and calculate the bone mineral density (BMD). The technique, however cannot distinguish between cortical and cancellous bone. The commonly scanned sites are the spine and femoral neck, with the estimated ratios of cortical-to-cancellous bone being 1:2 in the spine and 3:1 in the femoral neck. Thus, the measurements of the total BMD at these sites are more a reflection of trabecular bone density than measurements taken at the peripheral skeleton.

The BMD obtained can then be quantitatively translated into a numerical score, either a T-score (age independent) or a Z-score (age dependent). Osteoporosis is diagnosed when bone mineral density is less than or equal to 2.5 standard deviations below that of a healthy adult reference population. The WHO has established diagnostic guidelines based on the T-score (**Table 3.4-2**).

T-score	Interpretation
-1 and above	Normal
-1 to -2.5	Low bone mass
<-2.5	Osteoporosis
<-2.5 and fracture	Established osteoporosis

Table 3.4-2 Diagnostic guidelines for osteoporosis based on T-scores [1].

Common anatomical sites for measurements are the spine, hip, forearm, and calcaneum.

It should be noted that there are limitations in the use of T-scores in osteoporosis. Although the relative risk of vertebral fractures increases with osteoporosis, classification of osteoporosis by T-scores alone will miss patients with spine fractures (**Fig 3.4-3**). Fifty percent of women with vertebral fractures are not osteoporotic. BMD alone will miss one third of women needing treatment [11].

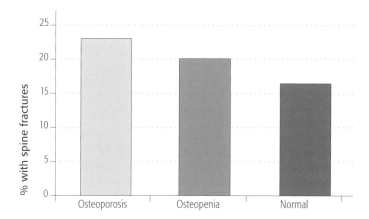

Fig 3.4-3 WHO classification by T-scores or BMD alone missing patients with factures [11].

While the T-score provides a useful numerical figure for the monitoring of osteoporosis, there are also other shortcomings that should be noted. There may be a slow response of the BMD to treatment. There is also a low signal-to-noise ratio and the increase in BMD may not be an adequate surrogate marker of efficacy of all treatments [12]. At present, the use of BMD together with biochemical markers of bone turnover (eg, type 1 collagen telopeptides) may help improve prediction of bone loss and fracture, as well as monitoring of therapy. There are also suggestions that when BMD is used with morphometric x-ray absorptiometry this helps improve the prediction of fractures.

Ultrasound attenuation and velocity

This method uses ultrasound waves to measure the bone trabecular pattern. Common anatomical sites for measurements include the calcaneum, patella, tibia, and forearm. In particular, the calcaneal quantitative ultrasound (QUS) is an alternative technique to DEXA for assessing bone mass. It measures both the velocity of sound (VOS) and broadband ultrasound attenuation. In constrast to DEXA, which solely measures bone mineral density, the QUS also gives additional information regarding the microstructural properties of cancellous bone [13–15]. While BMD is responsible for a significant proportion of bone strength, microarchitectural properties of trabecular bone (eg, strut number and thickness, trabeculae connectivity, orientation and spacing) are also important in determining fracture risk [16, 17]. Various studies have shown broadband ultrasound attenuation to be moderately correlated with BMD in the Caucasian population [17–19] and a more significant predictor of fracture risk than changes in the velocity of sound. For every one standard deviation (SD) change in broadband ultrasound attenuation, the risk of hip fracture doubles [20, 21].

The anatomical site (eg, the heel) is placed in the machine or a water bath and ultrasound waves pass through it to assess the bone quality (**Fig 4.3-4**). The reduction of ultrasound signal amplitude then allows measurement of bone quality. Osteoporotic bone, being less dense, absorbs less sound resulting in a reduced attenuation. Normal bone will therefore have a higher attenuation. The changes in broadband ultrasonic attenuation, typically over the range of 0.2–0.6 MHz, may then be used to estimate bone mineral density [22].

The obvious advantages of this method is that the heel/calcaneum is an easily accessible anatomical site. The costs involved

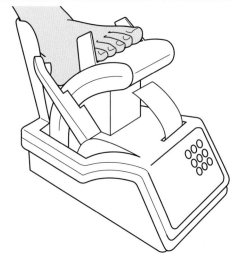

Fig 3.4-4 An ultrasound machine used for measuring BMD.

are also lower than that of DEXA and no radiation is involved. The machine is also small and portable, making it easily transportable and fixed office space unnecessary. While DEXA remains the gold standard for BMD measurement, DEXA as a population screening tool may not be cost effective [23] and is neither feasible in the UK [24] nor in the Asian population owing to limitations in resources. Ultrasound attenuation can be considered to be a more cost-effective alternative.

Some limitations of ultrasound attenuation include a greater population standard deviation compared to BMD [25]. In addition, the WHO criteria for BMD T-score values determined by DEXA may not be appropriate for interpretation by ultrasound attenuation owing to a different anatomical site with different rates of bone accretion and loss, together with a different measurement technology [26]. As a result, some studies recommend the use of an adjusted ultrasound attenuation score of –2.0 SD instead [25]. Finally, while some studies like that of Woon et al [27] have preliminary results to suggest that the ultrasound attenuation readings in an Asian population are similar to Caucasian values, further studies are still required to establish an appropriate reference range of ultrasonic attenuation for the Asian population before it can be used as an effective tool in the Asian population.

CT-based quantitative densitometry

Quantitative CT with a suitable software package enables the radiation absorption by different calcified tissues to be determined so that particular areas of interest (eg, the vertebral body) may be studied and analyzed. This technique measures true density and is expressed in g/cm^3 [28]. Tissue density is then compared with a calibration phantom.

Quantitative CT is principally used to determine trabecular bone density in the spine but can also be used to measure radial bone density [29]. Although a higher dose of radiation is required, quantitative CT is unique in that it can determine both bone density and distribution in three dimensions at any skeletal site. The bone density can be estimated separately in the trabecular and cortical bone components. It also allows extraosseous calcification to be distinguished, which would artificially increase the bone density reading as when measured with DEXA scanning (**Fig 3.4-5**) [30]. Trabecular diameter and intertrabecular spaces can be measured using a high resolution CT scan, and an abnormal trabecular pattern can be identified [31]. Its precision and accuracy of spinal measurements is within 2–4% and 5–10% respectively, and is regarded as having the best sensitivity and specificity for distinguishing patients with spinal osteoporosis from patients without it.

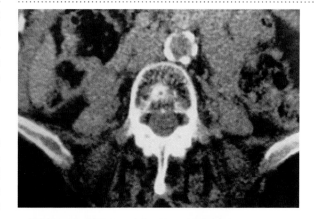

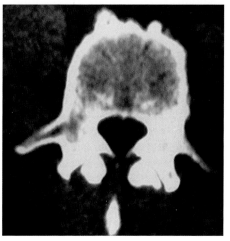

Fig 3.4-5 Two examples of extraosseous calcification which could affect DEXA readings but not CT quantitative densitometry.

Obesity

Obesity has become a global epidemic, especially for developed countries. It has been shown to be associated with chronic diseases and health issues like heart diseases, type II diabetes, hyperlipidemia, hypertension, sleep apnoea, certain cancers, and metabolic syndrome [32, 33]. Based on a WHO expert committee in 1995 [34], the body mass index (BMI) was recommended and various definitions of obesity were listed in 2000 (**Table 3.4-3**). The prevalence of individuals with a BMI of over 25 in the United States has risen from 44.3% in the late 1970s to 52.6% in the early 1990s, while in the same period individuals with a BMI of over 30 have risen from 13.4% to 21.2% [35]. The increased prevalence of overweight and obesity has resulted in an estimated USD 100 billion spent to treat obesity-related conditions annually in the USA, with the direct costs being approximately 5–10% of the total health care dollar spent annually [36].

Classification

Obesity is most simply and commonly measured by using the BMI. It was developed in the 19th century and in general is an accurate reflection of the percentage of body fat in the majority of the adult population. It is less accurate in individuals who may have a high percentage of muscle tissue (eg, body builders) or other complicated physiological states (eg, pregnancy).

The BMI is simply calculated by dividing the subject's weight in kilograms by the square of his or her height in meters:

BMI = weight (kg) / height (m) x height (m)

Alternatively, the BMI can be calculated in US customary units of pounds (lb) and inches (in):

BMI = weight (lb) x 703 / height (in) x height (in)

The most commonly used definition as provided by the WHO is listed below:

BMI	Classification
< 18.5	Underweight
18.5–24.9	Normal weight
25.0–29.9	Overweight
30.0–34.9	Class I obesity
35.0–39.9	Class II obesity
> 40.0	Class III obesity

Table 3.4-3 BMI classifications [37].

Relationship between BMI and disease

Studies have repeatedly shown a J-shaped relationship between BMI and relative risk and mortality [38–41], with emphasis on chronic diseases especially cardiovascular diseases. The point at which the health risk significantly increases, however, is subject to debate. Evidence suggests that there is a significant increase in health risk when the BMI is >25 kg/m^2, although there is also evidence that health risks may also increase at BMI level below 25 kg/m^2 [42–43]. Also, owing to the great diversity seen in the different peoples of the world, there is evidence to suggest that the associations with chronic diseases varies slightly from different geographic regions and ethnicities. In particular, in some Asian populations a specific BMI reflects a higher percentage of body fat than in Caucasian or European populations [44]. BMI cut-off points have been applied to Asian countries, and such cut-off points have been applied to trigger policy actions, to facilitate prevention programs, and to measure the effect of interventions (**Table 3.4-4** and **Fig 3.4-6**). Clinically, these values may be used to identify high-risk individuals for screening and for absolute risk assessments.

	Overweight		Obesity	
	Point analysis	Analysis of covariance	Point analysis	Analysis of covariance
China	24	25	29	30
Hong Kong	23	22	27	27
Indonesia	24	22	28	27
Japan	25	24	30	29
Singapore	22	23	27	27
Thailand (urban)	25	23	30	28
Thailand (rural)	27	25	31	30

Table 3.4-4 BMI cut-off points for overweight and obesity in Asian populations calculated by different methods [44].

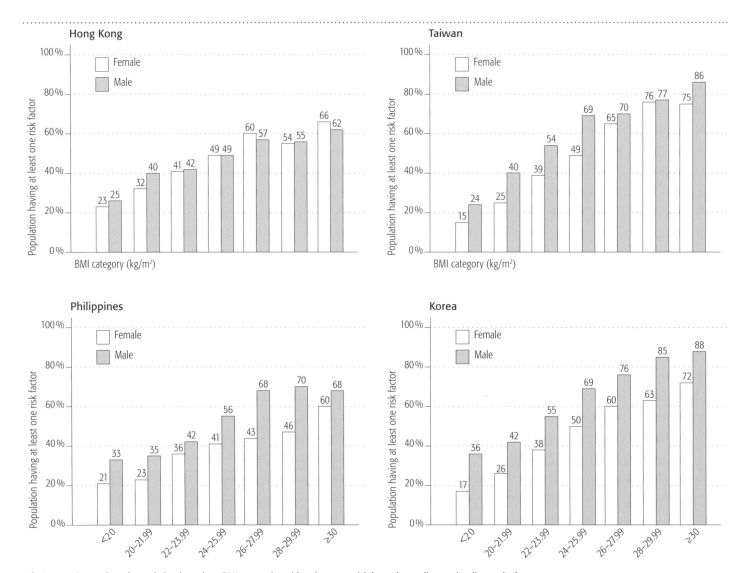

Fig 3.4-6 Proportion of population in various BMI categories with at least one risk factor for cardiovascular disease [44].

Measurement of body composition methods

More sophisticated methods of measuring body tissue composition, or body "fatness" are available. While there remains a good correlation between BMI and obesity, there are circumstances (eg, body builders, pregnancy, and highly fit athletes) where BMI measurements would be inaccurate. However, it should be noted that unlike the BMI method, these other methods provide no clear consensus on levels of body fatness that identify the point where morbidity and mortality significantly increase [41]. Therefore, apart from measuring body composition in response to treatment, it remains unclear how body fatness can be used until clinical standards of body compositions can be developed.

Methods to measure body composition can be subdivided into direct, indirect, and double indirect methods [45]. Direct methods measure the tissue component of interest, eg, in vivo neutron activation analysis (IVNAA). The elemental analysis of the body can be done using this method, after which the body tissue of interest can be calculated (eg, total body protein = 6.25 x total body nitrogen) [46]. IVNAA, however, is expensive and its availability is limited around the world.

Indirect methods

Indirect methods need to rely on assumptions that may not always be true. They rely on a 4-component model of minerals, protein, water, and body fat. The number of assumptions for such a 4-component model is small, and hence the possible bias is small. It is regarded as the best choice to measure body composition [47]. Indirect methods include:

- Densitometry
- Air displacement
- DEXA
- Near-infrared interactance (NIR) Futrex 5000

Densitometry (under water weighing or hydrostatic weighing)

Method: Based on Archimedes principle that when the body is submerged in water, a buoyancy counter effect would be equal to the mass of water displaced. Since fat is lighter and bone and muscle are more dense than water, by measuring the buoyancy effect the investigator is given an indication of the percentage of body fat. A larger amount of fat mass will make the body lighter in water.

Accuracy: This is a reasonably accurate test and, if performed correctly according to the guidelines, there is an approximate +/-1.5% margin of error. The accuracy will also depend on the patient's ability to exhale all the air from their lungs during a pre-test screening and during the test itself. Failure to do so will result in inaccuracy since air will make the body float more, and that will result in a miscalculation of the percentage of body fat.

Currently, this method is considered the gold standard in the measurement of percentage body fat. Also, repeat measures are usually shown to be consistent, so that the method can be reliably used to monitor a patient's progress. The test is also quite accurate. However, there are some drawbacks with this method. It can trigger anxiety in some patients as it requires them to be submerged under water for some time. The method also requires quite a lot of space for equipment. Testing is also time consuming and the final calculation of body fat does call for some in-depth knowledge.

Air displacement (Bod Pod)

Method: Based on the principle of water displacement, this is one of the newest methods of measuring body composition, using the Bod Pod developed by Life Measurement Instruments, Concord CA. Instead of using water displacement to measure body volume, the Bod Pod uses air displacement to measure body volume. Each test takes approximately 5–8 minutes.

Accuracy: With a reported margin of error of up to +/-3%, the accuracy of this method is again dependent on the correct performance of the test [48]. Slight movements or changes in breathing pattern will affect the readings. It is therefore important for a patient to remain still and to breathe normally. Currently, this method has significant advantages: it does not require a patient to get wet, it is relatively simple to operate, and measurement time is short. Its ease of use means that it is well suited for special population groups who may have difficulty with other methods of measurement (eg, children, the obese, the elderly, or the disabled). However, owing to the cost of the machine, this method is not widely available, making its use in population screening limited. It is currently mostly restricted to research laboratories and athletic facilities.

Dual energy x-ray absorptiometry (DEXA)

Method: DEXA, more commonly known for its use in measuring bone mineral density, is based on a 3-component model of body composition (body fat, muscle, and bone mineral). It uses two x-ray beams to measure body tissue based on the relative absorption of the different tissues of the body. The x-rays are then read off a computer software for the tissues and estimates for the whole body and regional body may be obtained.

Accuracy: Since DEXA takes into consideration the bone mineral element when estimating body fat and muscle (a 3-component model of body composition), it is regarded as more accurate and valid than methods that rely on a 2-component model of body composition (eg, hydrostatic weighing).

This method of measuring body composition is relatively quick (about 12 minutes) and no special preparation is required by the patient. The radiation dose required is also quite low. The main drawback of this method is in its costs.

Near-infrared interactance (NIR) Futrex 5000

Method: This method of measuring body tissue composition is based on the principles of light absorption, reflectance, and near-infrared spectroscopy. It uses a computerized spectrophotometer that has a scanner and probe. The probe is first placed on the selected body site. It then emits an infrared light that passes through the tissues and is then reflected back. Density measures are obtained and incorporated into the manufacturer's prediction equations and a digital readout of percentage body fat and lean tissue is displayed.

Accuracy: This method of assessing body fat is not the most accurate [49]. Skin fold measurement was found to be more accurate than NIR when hydrostatic weighing was used as the measurement criterion. NIR was found to underestimate body fat by more than 4% in subjects with greater than 30% fat and overestimates body fat by 4% in subjects with less than 8% body fat.

NIR is generally safe, noninvasive, fast, and convenient. It is also fairly inexpensive. However, as stated above, its accuracy is not very good.

Double indirect method

Double indirect methods rely on a statistical association between easily measurable body variables and a measure of body composition, usually obtained through an indirect method. As such, these are no more than predictions and bias does occur at an individual level and population level.

Common methods in this category are the following:

- Skin fold measurements
- Bioelectric impedance
- Waist circumference

Skin fold measurements

Method: A skin fold caliper (eg, Lange or Harpenden) is used to measure subcutaneous tissue in specific areas of the body. The Lange skin fold caliper is the one more widely used in schools, colleges, and fitness centers, while the Harpenden is the standard caliper used in research. This is probably the most widely used method. The 7-site skin fold measurement includes the chest, triceps brachii, subscapular, axilla, suprailiac, abdomen, and thigh. A shortened 3-site skin fold measurement differs slightly for men and women, due to the physiological differences between the sexes. The 3-site skin fold measurement for men includes the chest, abdomen, and thigh, while that for the women includes the triceps brachii, suprailiac, and thigh.

This method requires the proper definition of anatomical landmarks such that results are consistently reproducible. The measurement technique also needs to be reproducible. In general, the Harpenden calipers are calibrated to 40 mm in 0.2 mm divisions, and have a compression of $10 \, g/mm^2$. An anthropometric tape is required to locate the skin sites and it should not be nonextensible but flexible, should be no wider than 7 mm, and should have a blank area of at least 3 cm before the zero line [50].

The skin fold is raised by the left hand in such a manner that the thumb points downward and the back of the hand is in full view of the measurer. The fold should be elevated slightly away from the body in order to give the calipers a better grip and reduce the chances of them slipping. For left-handed measurers, it is important for consistency that the calipers and the way the skin fold is raised should be similar to a right-handed measurer performing the measurement.

The calipers should be placed about 1 cm between the near edge of the fingers and the nearest edge of the calipers face. The calipers should also not be applied too deeply (where it might exaggerate the skin fold) or superficially (where it might slip off). In general, measurements are taken on the right side of the body unless there is a specific study or reason to perform otherwise.

Accuracy: If each of the tests are performed according to the recommended guidelines, there will be a +/-3% margin of error.

This method of body fat measurement is operator dependent, but easy to use once the skill has been mastered. It does not require a lot of time and is noninvasive. It is also an inexpensive method of measuring body fat. It, however, may not be suitable for those who are very obese or very lean, as the technical sources of error would be highest in such cases. As it is a measure of subcutaneous fat, skin fold measurement only serves as a prediction of the amount of total fat of an individual.

Bioelectric impedence

Method: Bioelectric impedence is based on the principle that different tissues in the body have different conductivity to an electric current, with fat being a poor conductor of electricity. It involves having a patient stand barefoot on two metal plates, where an undetectably low electric current is sent up one leg and down the other. Since fat impedes the flow of current more than lean tissue, by measuring the amount of resistance to the electric current, the impedance machine is able to estimate the amount of body fat.

Accuracy: There is a +/-3% margin of error. However, the accuracy of bioelectric impedence depends on several patient-related factors. Patients should follow the protocol below:

- Abstain from eating and drinking within 4 hours of the test
- Avoid exercising within 12 hours of the test
- Void the bladder completely prior to testing
- No alcohol consumption 48 hours before the test
- Avoid taking diuretics prior to testing

Bioelectric impedence is quick (lasting less than 1 minute) and requires little or no technical knowledge from the operator or patient. The unit for testing is easily transportable and essentially just requires an electric outlet and the machine itself. However, owing to the relatively large number of variables, this method tends to have a higher error range. There is also the tendency for the test to overestimate lean people and underestimate obese ones.

Waist circumference and waist-hip ratio
By using an anthropometric tape (which should be non-extensible but flexible) direct measurements of the waist circumference or the ratio of the waist-to-hip circumferences can be simply obtained. A waist circumference of more than 102 cm in men and 88 cm in women and a waist-hip ratio of more than 0.9 in men and 0.85 in women are all taken as measures of central obesity [51]. Intraabdominal or visceral fat has a particularly strong correlation with cardiovascular disease. Women with abdominal obesity have a cardiovascular risk similar to men [52], and in general, waist circumference had a better correlation to metabolic syndrome than the BMI [53].

Summary

There is a clear clinical importance to structural body composition measurement values. In cases of morbid obesity, significant weight loss is often advised prior to proceeding with an elective procedure. When instrumenting the axial or appendicular skeleton, consideration of bone mineral density is highly advisable as it may later influence management. It is also important to note that there may be variability in how the T-score is generated and interpreted depending on the instruments and personnel. Surgeons may choose supplemental immobilization, instrumentation augmentation with cement, or may choose to forego instrumentation altogether. Familiarity with the body composition measurement techniques and their respective clinical translations are of great importance for surgical decision making.

References

1. **World Health Organization** (1994) Assessment of fracture risk and its application to screening for postmenopausal osteoporosis. Report of a WHO Study Group. *World Health Organ Tech Rep Ser* 843; 1–129.
2. **International Osteoporosis Foundation** (2005) International Osteoporosis Foundation (IOF). www.osteofound.org.
3. **No authors listed** (1984) Consensus conference: Osteoporosis. *Jama;* 252:799–802.
4. **Dennison E, Cooper C** (2000) Epidemiology of osteoporotic fractures. *Horm Res;* 1:58–63.
5. **Nordin BEC** (1984) *Osteoporosis: Metabolic bone and stone disease.* Churchhill Livingstone: Edinburgh.
6. **Lindsay R** (1988) *Pathogenesis, detection and prevention of postmenopausal osteoporosis.* Blackwell Scientific Publications: Oxford.
7. **Lippuner K, von Overbeck J, Perrelet R, et al** (1997) Incidence and direct medical costs of hospitalizations due to osteoporotic fractures in Switzerland. *Osteoporosis Int;* 7:414–425
8. **Riggs BL, Melton LJ, 3rd** (1995) The worldwide problem of osteoporosis: insights afforded by epidemiology. *Bone;* 17:505S–511S.
9. **Schott AM, Cormier C, Hans D, et al** (1998) How hip and whole-body bone mineral density predict hip fracture in elderly women: the EPIDOS Prospective Study. *Osteoporos Int;* 8:247–254.
10. **Marshall D, Johnell O, Wedel H** (1996) Meta–analysis of how well measures of bone mineral density predict occurrence of osteoporotic fractures. *BMJ;* 312:1254–1259.
11. **Greenspan SL, von Stetten E, Emond SK, et al** (2001) Instant vertebral assessment: a noninvasive dual X-ray absorptiometry technique to avoid misclassification and clinical mismanagement of osteoporosis. *J Clin Densitom;* 4:373–380.
12. **Garnero P, Delmas PD** (2004) Noninvasive techniques for assessing skeletal changes in inflammatory arthritis: bone biomarkers. *Curr Opin Rheumatol;* 16:428–434.
13. **Gluer CC, Vahlensieck M, Faulkner KG, et al** (1992) Site-matched calcaneal measurements of broad-band ultrasound attenuation and single X-ray absorptiometry: do they measure different skeletal properties? *J Bone Miner Res;* 7:1071–1079.
14. **Kaufman JJ, Einhorn TA** (1993) Ultrasound assessment of bone. *J Bone Miner Res;* 8:517–525.
15. **Gluer CC, Wu CY, Genant HK** (1993) Broadband ultrasound attenuation signals depend on trabecular orientation: an in vitro study. *Osteoporos Int;* 3:185–191.
16. **Hayes WC, Piazza SJ, Zysset PK** (1991) Biomechanics of fracture risk prediction of the hip and spine by quantitative computed tomography. *Radiol Clin North Am;* 29:1–18.
17. **Ensrud KE, Black DM, Palermo L, et al** (1997) Treatment with alendronate prevents fractures in women at highest risk: results from the Fracture Intervention Trial. *Arch Intern Med;* 157:2617–2624.
18. **Faulkner KG, McClung MR, Coleman LJ, et al** (1994) Quantitative ultrasound of the heel: correlation with densitometric measurements at different skeletal sites. *Osteoporos Int;* 4:42–47.
19. **Hans D, Njeh CF, Genant HK, et al** (1998) Quantitative ultrasound in bone status assessment. *Rev Rhum Engl Ed;* 65:489–498.
20. **Porter RW, Miller CG, Grainger D, et al** (1990) Prediction of hip fracture in elderly women: a prospective study. *BMJ;* 301:638–641.
21. **Pluijm SM, Graafmans WC, Bouter LM, et al** (1999) Ultrasound measurements for the prediction of osteoporotic fractures in elderly people. *Osteoporos Int;* 9:550–556.
22. **Langton CM, Njeh CF** (2008) The measurement of broadband ultrasonic attenuation in cancellous bone—a review of the science and technology. *IEEE Trans Ultrason Ferroelectr Freq Control;* 55:1546–1554.
23. **Langton CM, Ballard PA, Bennett DK, et al** (1997) A comparison of the sensitivity and specificity of calcaneal ultrasound measurements with clinical criteria for bone densitometry (DEXA) referral. *Clin Rheumatol;* 16:117–118.
24. **Fogelman I** (1999) Screening for osteoporosis. No point until we have resolved issues about long term treatment. *BMJ;* 319:1148–1149.
25. **Frost ML, Blake GM, Fogelman I** (1999) Contact quantitative ultrasound: an evaluation of precision, fracture discrimination, age-related bone loss and applicability of the WHO criteria. *Osteoporos Int;* 10:441–449.
26. **Greenspan SL, Maitland-Ramsey L, Myers E** (1996) Classification of osteoporosis in the elderly is dependent on site-specific analysis. *Calcif Tissue Int;* 58:409–414.
27. **Woon CY, Chong KC, Lim YM, et al** (2006) Broadband Ultrasound Attenuation compared with dual energy X-ray absorptiometry in screening for osteoporosis in an Asian population. *J Orthopaedics;* 3:e16.
28. **Banks LM, Stevenson JC** (1990) *Developments in computerized axial tomography scanning and its use in bone disease measurement.* New techniques in metabolic bone disease. Wright: London.
29. **Grampp S, Lang P, Jergas M, et al** (1995) Assessment of the skeletal status by peripheral quantitative computed tomography of the forearm: short-term precision in vivo and comparison to dual X-ray absorptiometry. *J Bone Miner Res;* 10:1566–1576.
30. **Sandor T, Felsenberg D, Kalender WA, et al** (1992) Compact and trabecular components of the spine using quantitative computed tomography. *Calcif Tissue Int;* 50:502–506.
31. **Mundinger A, Wiesmeier B, Dinkel E, et al** (1993) Quantitative image analysis of vertebral body architecture—improved diagnosis in osteoporosis based on high-resolution computed tomography. *Br J Radiol;* 66:209–213.

32. **Grundy SM** (2004) Obesity, metabolic syndrome, and cardiovascular disease. *J Clin Endocrinol Metab;* 89:2595–2600.

33. **Haslam DW, James WP** (2005) Obesity. *Lancet;* 366:1197–209.

34. **World Health Organization** (1995) Physical Status: the use and interpretation of anthropometry. Report of a WHO Expert Consultation. *World Health Organ Tech Rep Ser* 854; 1–452

35. **Flegal KM, Carroll MD, Kuczmarski RJ, et al** (1998) Overweight and obesity in the United States: prevalence and trends, 1960–1994. *Int J Obes Relat Metab Disord;* 22:39–47.

36. **Wolf AM, Colditz GA** (1998) Current estimates of the economic cost of obesity in the United States. *Obes Res;* 6:97–106.

37. **World Health Organization** (2000) Obesity: preventing and managing the global epidemic. Report on a WHO Consultation. *World Health Organ Tech Rep Ser* 894; 1–253

38. **Barrett-Connor EL** (1985) Obesity, atherosclerosis, and coronary artery disease. *Ann Intern Med;* 103:1010–1019.

39. **Drenick EJ, Bale GS, Seltzer F, et al** (1980) Excessive mortality and causes of death in morbidly obese men. *Jama;* 243:443–445.

40. **Larsson B, Bjorntorp P, Tibblin G** (1981) The health consequences of moderate obesity. *Int J Obes;* 5:97–116.

41. **Jakicic JM, Clark K, Coleman E, et al** (2001) American College of Sports Medicine position stand. Appropriate intervention strategies for weight loss and prevention of weight regain for adults. *Med Sci Sports Exerc;* 33:2145–2156.

42. **Manson JE, Willett WC, Stampfer MJ, et al** (1995) Body weight and mortality among women. *N Engl J Med;* 333:677–685.

43. **Stevens J, Cai J, Pamuk ER, et al** (1998) The effect of age on the association between body-mass index and mortality. *N Engl J Med;* 338:1–7.

44. **World Health Organization** (2004) Appropriate body-mass index for Asian populations and its implications for policy and intervention strategies. *Lancet;* 363:157–163.

45. **Deurenberg P** (1992) The assessment of body composition: use and misuse. *Annual Report Nestle Foundation;* 35–72.

46. **Wang ZM, Pierson RN, Jr., Heymsfield SB** (1992) The five-level model: a new approach to organizing body-composition research. *Am J Clin Nutr;* 56:19–28.

47. **Heymsfield SB, Waki M** (1991) Body composition in humans: advances in the development of multicompartment chemical models. *Nutr Rev;* 49:97–108.

48. **McCrory MA, Gomez TD, Bernauer EM, et al** (1995) Evaluation of a new air displacement plethysmograph for measuring human body composition. *Med Sci Sports Exerc;* 27:1686–1691.

49. **McLean KP, Skinner JS** (1992) Validity of Futrex-5000 for body composition determination. *Med Sci Sports Exerc;* 24:253–258.

50. **Norton KI, Marfell-Jones M, Whittingham N, et al** (2000) *Anthropometric assessment protocols.* Human Kinetics.

51. **Yusuf S, Hawken S, Ounpuu S, et al** (2004) Effect of potentially modifiable risk factors associated with myocardial infarction in 52 countries (the INTERHEART study): case-control study. *Lancet;* 364:937–952.

52. **Larsson B, Bengtsson C, Bjorntorp P, et al** (1992) Is abdominal body fat distribution a major explanation for the sex difference in the incidence of myocardial infarction? The study of men born in 1913 and the study of women, Goteborg, Sweden. *Am J Epidemiol;* 135:266–273.

53. **Janssen I, Katzmarzyk PT, Ross R** (2004) Waist circumference and not body mass index explains obesity-related health risk. *Am J Clin Nutr;* 79:379–384.

3.4.1   Osteoporosis

1   Bone mineral density (BMD) using quantitative computed tomography (QCT)

Description

Measurement of trabecular BMD in single transverse CT slices at the lumbar midvertebral level and at the forearm.

Interpretation

10–20% of change of cortex thickness can be measured accurately.

Clinical relevance

Modest radiation exposures (100 μSv). High precision (1–2% for BMD of the spine, hip and radius); nearly instant availability of data (seconds to minutes); widespread access and minimal user interaction. Cortical and trabecular bone can be analyzed separately.

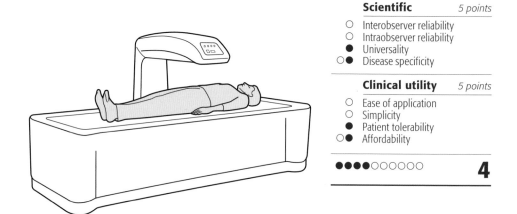

Fig 3.4.1-1

Reliability

Population tested in	Interobserver reliability	Intraobserver reliability
Not tested		

2   Bone mineral density (BMD) using dual energy x-ray absorptiometry (DEXA)

Description
BMD measures are obtained in the posteroanterior spine and the hip.

Interpretation
Osteoporosis is defined in terms of a T-score below −2.5 and osteopenia when the T-score is between −2.5 and −1.

Clinical relevance
The reference method to measure BMD allows accurate diagnosis of osteoporosis, estimation of fracture risk, and monitoring of patients undergoing treatments. Requires detailed attention to proper positioning and analyses of the results. Exposure to radiation.

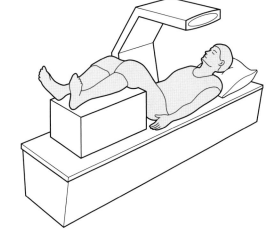

Fig 3.4.1-2

SCORING   *10 total points*

Scientific   *5 points*
- ○ Interobserver reliability
- ○ Intraobserver reliability
- ● Universality
- ○● Disease specificity

Clinical utility   *5 points*
- ● Ease of application
- ● Simplicity
- ● Patient tolerability
- ●● Affordability

●●●●●●●○○○   **7**

Reliability

Population tested in	Interobserver reliability	Intraobserver reliability
Not tested		

3   Density and microarchitectural properties of bone, either cortical or cancellous bone using quantitative ultrasound (QUS)

Description

It can be performed using ultrasound measurements of the calcaneus, patella, tibia, phalanges, radius, and metatarsal, with a range of techniques including transmission and semi-reflection or axial transmission mode ultrasound.

Interpretation

Sensitive to age-related, pubertal stage, and menopause-related changes in bone. It is a good predictor or discriminator of hip or nonspinal fractures. Studies have found QUS to be sensitive to clinical risk factors for osteoporosis and secondary causes of osteoporosis. QUS may be of use for the prediction of those at risk of future fracture in areas where there is limited availability of DEXA.

Clinical relevance

QUS has demonstrated limited use in the monitoring of patients undergoing treatment, primarily due to its poor precision in comparison with DEXA, leading to long time intervals being required. Its precision is generally reported to be poorer than that of DEXA in detecting changes in bone.

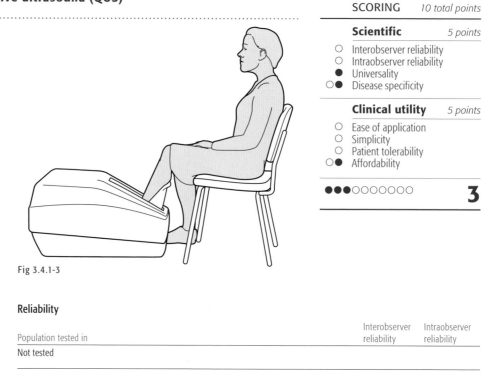

Fig 3.4.1-3

Reliability

Population tested in	Interobserver reliability	Intraobserver reliability
Not tested		

SCORING	10 total points

Scientific	5 points
○ Interobserver reliability	
○ Intraobserver reliability	
● Universality	
○● Disease specificity	

Clinical utility	5 points
○ Ease of application	
○ Simplicity	
○ Patient tolerability	
○● Affordability	

●●●○○○○○○○   **3**

4   Singh index [1]

Description
Evaluates the trabeculae in the upper end of the femur, which are arranged along the lines of compression and tension stresses produced in the bone during weight bearing, visualized in plain roentgenograms of the hip region.

Interpretation
Grade 6: All the normal trabeculae groups are visible and the upper end of the femur seems to be completely occupied by cancellous bone.

Grade 5: The structure of the principal compressive and tensile trabeculae is accentuated. Ward's triangle appears prominently.

Grade 4: Principal tensile trabeculae are markedly reduced in number but can still be traced from the lateral cortex to the upper part of the femoral neck.

Grade 3: There is a break in the continuity of the principal tensile trabeculae opposite the great trochanter. This grade means definite osteoporosis.

Grade 2: Only the principal compressive trabeculae stand out prominently; the others have been resorbed more or less completely.

Grade 1: Even the principal compressive trabeculae are markedly reduced in number and are no longer prominent.

Clinical relevance
This tool is easy to use for qualitative assessment of bone mineral density utilizing an AP x-ray of the hip.

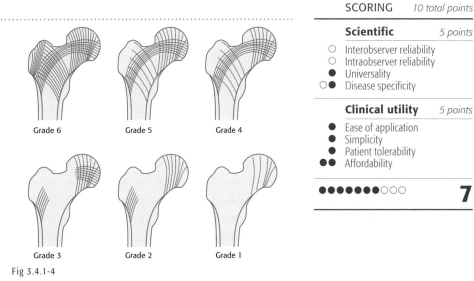

Grade 6   Grade 5   Grade 4

Grade 3   Grade 2   Grade 1

Fig 3.4.1-4

Reliability

Population tested in	Interobserver reliability	Intraobserver reliability
Not tested		

SCORING   *10 total points*

Scientific   *5 points*
- ○ Interobserver reliability
- ○ Intraobserver reliability
- ● Universality
- ○● Disease specificity

Clinical utility   *5 points*
- ● Ease of application
- ● Simplicity
- ● Patient tolerability
- ●● Affordability

●●●●●●●○○○   **7**

References:
1 **Singh M, Nagrath AR, Maini PS** (1970) Changes in trabecular pattern of the upper end of the femur as an index of osteoporosis. *J Bone Joint Surg Am;* 52:457–467.

3.4.2   Obesity

1   Skin fold measurements

Description

A skin fold caliper (eg, Lange or Harpenden) is used to measure subcutaneous tissue in seven specific areas of the body:

- Triceps brachii
- Biceps brachii
- Subscapularis
- Supraspinatus
- Lower abdomen
- Thigh
- Calf

The Lange skin fold caliper is more widely used in schools, colleges, and fitness centers, while the Harpenden is the standard caliper used in research. This is probably the most widely used method.

Interpretation

Differentiated into five categories (approximation):

- 40–80—Excellent
- 70–90—Good
- 90–110—Average
- 110–140—Below average
- >140—Poor

Clinical relevance

Skinfold thickness can allow for prospective intraindividual assessments. There are gender-specific variations. There is a lack of reliability with morbid obesity.

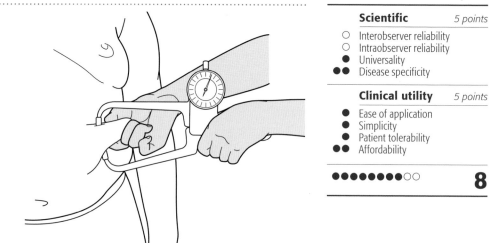

Fig 3.4.2-1

Reliability

Population tested in	Interobserver reliability	Intraobserver reliability
Not tested		

SCORING	10 total points
Scientific	5 points

- ○ Interobserver reliability
- ○ Intraobserver reliability
- ● Universality
- ●● Disease specificity

Clinical utility	5 points

- ● Ease of application
- ● Simplicity
- ● Patient tolerability
- ●● Affordability

●●●●●●●●○○   **8**

2 Densitometry

SCORING   *10 total points*

Description

When the body is submerged in water, a buoyancy counter effect would be equal to the mass of water displaced. Fat is lighter and bone and muscle are more dense than water.

Interpretation

Measuring the buoyancy effect would give the investigator an indication of the percentage of body fat. A larger amount of fat mass will make the body lighter in water.

Body fat percentage is then calculated.

Clinical relevance

Body fat percentages are more relevant for obesity assessment and management. The procedure is expensive, time consuming, nonportable, and comes with a fear of infection.

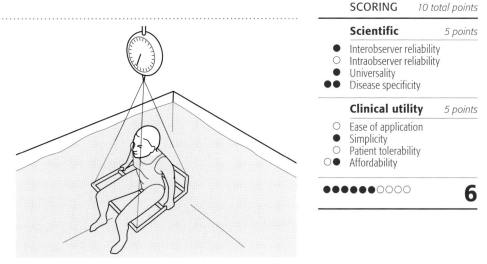

Fig 3.4.2-2

Scientific *5 points*

● Interobserver reliability
○ Intraobserver reliability
● Universality
●● Disease specificity

Clinical utility *5 points*

○ Ease of application
● Simplicity
○ Patient tolerability
○● Affordability

●●●●●●○○○○   **6**

Reliability

Population tested in	Interobserver reliability	Intraobserver reliability
Densitometry and x-rays of patients with varying severities of vertebral deformities (N = 205) evaluated by two observers [1]	+ Grade 2 or higher severity - < Grade 2 or lower severity	NA

References:
1. Schousboe JT, Debold CR (2006) Reliability and accuracy of vertebral fracture assessment with densitometry compared to radiography in clinical practice. *Osteoporos Int;* 17:281–289.

3   Bioelectric impedance

Description
Different tissues in the body have different conductivity to an electric current, with fat being a poor conductor of electricity. It involves having a subject stand barefoot on two metal plates. An undetectably low electric current is sent up one leg and down the other. Fat impedes the flow of current more than lean tissue.

Interpretation
By measuring the amount of resistance to the electric current, the impedance machine is able to estimate the amount of body fat.

Clinical relevance
After initial limitations due to lack of reliability, this modality is now considered more reliable but lacks standardized methodology and quality control.

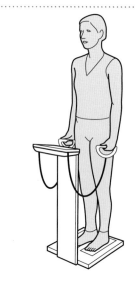

Fig 3.4.2-3

SCORING   *10 total points*

Scientific   *5 points*
○ Interobserver reliability
○ Intraobserver reliability
● Universality
●● Disease specificity

Clinical utility   *5 points*
● Ease of application
● Simplicity
● Patient tolerability
○● Affordability

●●●●●●●○○○   **7**

Reliability

Population tested in	Interobserver reliability	Intraobserver reliability
Not tested		

4   Waist circumference and waist-hip ratio

Description
Anthropometric tape (which should be nonextensible but flexible) allows for measurements of the waist circumference or the ratio of the waist to hip circumference.

Interpretation
A waist circumference of more than 102 cm in men and 88 cm in women and a waist-hip ratio of more than 0.9 in men and 0.85 in women are taken as measures of central obesity.

Clinical relevance
Positive association with metabolic syndrome, type-2 diabetes, hypertension, and cardiovascular disease has been established.

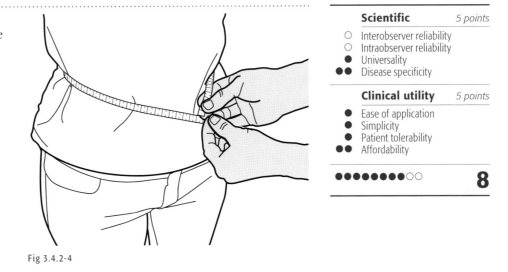

Fig 3.4.2-4

Reliability

Population tested in	Interobserver reliability	Intraobserver reliability
Not tested		

SCORING   *10 total points*

Scientific   *5 points*
○ Interobserver reliability
○ Intraobserver reliability
● Universality
●● Disease specificity

Clinical utility   *5 points*
● Ease of application
● Simplicity
● Patient tolerability
●● Affordability

●●●●●●●●○○   **8**

5   Air displacement plethysmography (ADP)

Description
Based on the principle of water displacement. Instead of using water displacement to measure body volume, the Bod Pod uses air displacement to measure body volume and allows estimates of fat mass and free fat mass.

Interpretation
Determination of visceral adipose tissue with ADP is considered valid and reliable and expressed as a percentage with a range of 4–45%.

Clinical relevance
Population-based testing. Individual health status assessments. Expensive, nonportable, and service intensive.

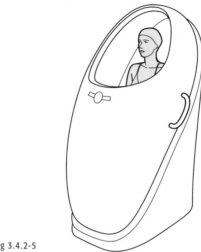

Fig 3.4.2-5

SCORING   *10 total points*

Scientific   *5 points*
○ Interobserver reliability
○ Intraobserver reliability
● Universality
●● Disease specificity

Clinical utility   *5 points*
○ Ease of application
○ Simplicity
○ Patient tolerability
○○ Affordability

●●●○○○○○○○   **3**

Reliability

Population tested in	Interobserver reliability	Intraobserver reliability
Not tested		

6 Dual energy x-ray absorptiometry (DEXA)

Description

DEXA, more commonly known for its use in measuring bone mineral density, is based on a 3-component model of body composition: body fat, muscle, and bone mineral. It uses two x-ray energies to measure body tissue based on the relative absorption of the different tissues of the body. The x-rays are then read by computer software for the tissues and estimates of the whole body and regional body may be obtained.

Scientific *5 points*

○ Interobserver reliability
○ Intraobserver reliability
● Universality
●● Disease specificity

Clinical utility *5 points*

● Ease of application
● Simplicity
● Patient tolerability
○○ Affordability

●●●●●●●○○○　　**6**

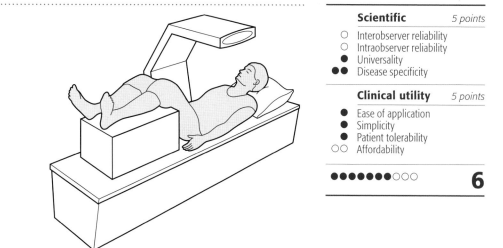

Fig 3.4.2-6

Interpretation

This test shows the percentage of body fat.

Clinical relevance

Radiation and resource-intensive application. Not widely used.

Reliability

Population tested in	Interobserver reliability	Intraobserver reliability
Not tested		

7   Infrared

SCORING   *10 total points*

Description
Uses light absorption, reflectance, and near-infrared spectroscopy.
A computerized spectrophotometer is used with a scanner and probe.
The probe is first placed on the selected body site. The infrared light is reflected by muscle and absorbed by fat.
Density measures are obtained and incorporated into the manufacturer's prediction equations and a digital readout of percentage body fat and lean tissue is displayed.

This technique was developed by the US Department of Agriculture for meat quality control.

Interpretation
Percentage of body fat to muscle.

Clinical relevance
This device has not been approved by the US Food and Drug Administration. Single manufacture only. While rapid and noninvasive, this method has produced inconsistent results due to different skin absorption.

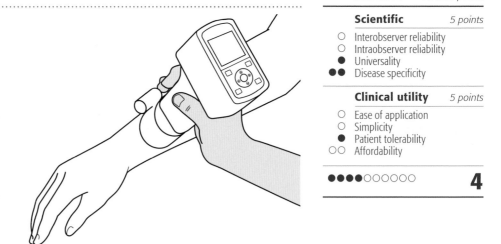

Fig 3.4.2-7

Scientific   5 points

○   Interobserver reliability
○   Intraobserver reliability
●   Universality
●●   Disease specificity

Clinical utility   5 points

○   Ease of application
○   Simplicity
●   Patient tolerability
○○   Affordability

●●●●○○○○○○   **4**

Reliability

Population tested in	Interobserver reliability	Intraobserver reliability
Not tested		

8 MRI

Description
Conventional MRI.

Interpretation
Qualitative assessment of the relative proportion of adipose tissue.

Clinical relevance
Cost prohibitive.

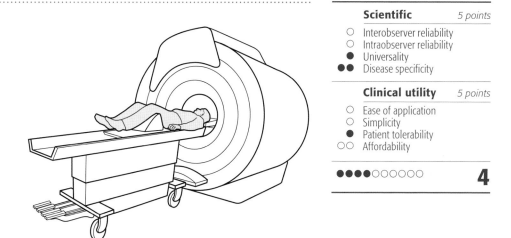

Fig 3.4.2-8

Reliability

Population tested in	Interobserver reliability	Intraobserver reliability
Not tested		

SCORING   *10 total points*

Scientific   *5 points*
- ○ Interobserver reliability
- ○ Intraobserver reliability
- ● Universality
- ●● Disease specificity

Clinical utility   *5 points*
- ○ Ease of application
- ○ Simplicity
- ● Patient tolerability
- ○○ Affordability

●●●●○○○○○○   **4**

9   CT

Description
Conventional CT.

Interpretation
Qualitative assessment of the relative
proportion of adipose tissue.

Clinical relevance
Radiation.

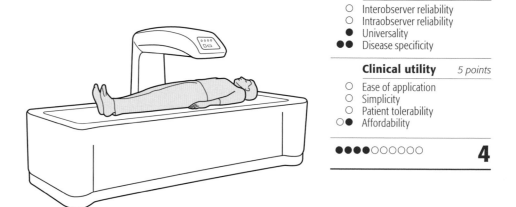

Fig 3.4.2-9

SCORING   *10 total points*

Scientific   *5 points*
○ Interobserver reliability
○ Intraobserver reliability
● Universality
●● Disease specificity

Clinical utility   *5 points*
○ Ease of application
○ Simplicity
○ Patient tolerability
○● Affordability

●●●●○○○○○○   **4**

Reliability

Population tested in	Interobserver reliability	Intraobserver reliability
Not tested		

4   Laboratory measurements
4.1 Blood/urine/plasma/serum measurements

4 Laboratory measurements

4.1 Blood/urine/plasma/serum measurements

Introduction

The work up of pathological or traumatic spinal disease includes laboratory testing targeted at discovering the underlying causes of spinal disease, such as infection, rheumatological disorders, cancer, and toxicology. In addition, tests may be indicated to detect conditions that affect recommended treatment, surgical wound healing, and—in the case of patients undergoing surgical therapy—perioperative risks.

Underlying causes of spinal disease

Nutrition and metabolism

Nutritional and metabolic issues have implications for spinal disease, deformity and pain, and for postoperative issues, such as wound healing and infection [1]. The basic nutritional work up should include serum protein and albumin. **Table 4.1-1** shows an extensive work-up for patients with metabolic bone disease.

Metabolic bone disease	
Primary hyperparathyroidism	• Parathyroid hormone levels (PTH) • Serum calcium: total, free ionized • Phosphate: serum and urine • Alkaline phosphatase • Serum bone-specific alkaline phosphatase • Tubular reabsorption of phosphate • Bone mineral metabolism • Serum chloride-phosphate ratio • Urine cyclic AMP
Vitamin D deficiency (rickets, osteomalacia, osteoporosis)	• Serum vitamin D (25-hydroxyvitamin D) levels
Hyperthyroid	• Thyroid function studies: TSH, T3, free T4
Megaloblastic anemia	• Serum B12 levels
Osteoporosis	• Procollagen, urine bone markers (eg N-telopeptide), serum telopeptides, urine hydroxyproline

Table 4.1-1 Work-up for patients with metabolic bone disease.

Infection

Infection continues to be a serious and common cause of spinal disease, as well as a cause of postoperative complications [2]. Infectious diseases commonly presenting in the spine or its surrounding tissues include *Staphylococcus aureus*, *Mycobacterium tuberculosis*, and *Brucella spp* (common in Mediterranean countries). Diagnosis is supported by laboratory data but can be confirmed only by isolation of the causative organism or histological evidence (blood culture or tissue biopsy), or suggestive serological testing [3].

Skin testing for tuberculosis should be considered in populations with an increased risk for tuberculosis, such as patients with suppressed immunity, homeless individuals, alcoholics, prisoners, intravenous drug users, or immigrants from sub-Saharan Africa, the Indian subcontinent, and southeast Asia [4].

HIV testing may be useful in detecting causes of immunocompromise and directing further search for infectious agents as an etiology of spinal pathology. HIV serology and subsequent cluster of differentiation 4 (CD4) testing are reasonable starting tests if HIV related pathology is suspected. While some practitioners have adopted the practice of screening all surgical patients for HIV, presumably in order to affect operating room precautions, this practice is specifically not recommended. Universal precautions are the standard of practice for all surgical patients. Screening for HIV is not only expensive, but may be misleading. Negative HIV tests can occur in the early stages of HIV infection, when positive antibody titers have not yet developed, and viral load is at its highest—ie, when the patient is actually highly infectious.

In patients who have current infections, or for whom infection needs to be ruled out, white cell count (WCC), erythrocyte sedimentation rate, and C-reactive protein [3] tests are helpful, in addition to establishing the nutritional status of the patient. Preoperative blood cultures serology for suspected organisms and intraoperative tissue/bone cultures are advisable.

Rheumatological disorders

Rheumatological disorders leading to spinal pain and deformity include rheumatoid arthritis, ankylosing spondylitis, and osteoarthritis. Patients with rheumatological arthritis present with multiple complications, including wound breakdown, infection, and pseudoarthritis [5]. Care must be taken to appropriately diagnose and optimize treatment prior to surgery. Appropriate tests include rheumatoid factor, antinuclear antibody, and human leukocyte antigen (HLA) testing. However, the results of these tests, positive or negative, must be interpreted in the context of a full rheumatological work-up as these disorders can be present in the absence of positive serology. Additional tests to consider are serum IgA, lipid levels, amyloid A, and cyclic citrullinated peptide (CCP) antibody testing.

Toxicology

Toxicology tests can identify potential toxic causes of spinal disease, such as iron and aluminum toxicity. Serum toxicology screening in certain cases may reveal overuse of narcotic medication, either as a result of polypharmacy or as a result of medication-seeking behavior. Such discoveries may help direct the appropriate triage of a patient presenting with spinal pain and other symptoms so that they can be referred to the appropriate nonsurgical healthcare providers.

Oncologic diseases affecting the spine

Most tumors presenting in the spine are due to metastatic disease. Metastasis to the spine is seen in 5–10% of cancer patients with a majority of the tumor types being lung, breast, and lymphoma [6]. These patients present with spinal compression as the first sign of neoplastic disease, and testing is usually first directed at x-ray evaluation.

Other conditions that commonly affect the spine include prostate and renal cancer, and multiple myeloma. Serum prostate specific antigen (PSA) levels may be useful in evaluating treatment of prostate cancer. Laboratory studies that may be helpful at ruling out multiple myeloma include serum protein and urine protein electrophoresis [7].

Preoperative laboratory evaluation includes tests to confirm normal hematological, hepatic, renal, and coagulation function in patients when abnormalities of these issues are suspected. Studies have failed to show a significant value in performing routine preoperative laboratory tests on healthy patients.

Preoperative coagulation screening prothrombin time (PT), partial thromboplastin time (PTT), and international normalized ratio (INR) may be useful if the patient's history or physical exam suggests the presence of a bleeding disorder. However, these tests are in general not useful as a preoperative screening device in normal patients, even when the surgery is expected to be extensive. Answers to the following questions can discern whether or not preoperative coagulation screening is warranted:

- Has the patient been diagnosed with a bleeding disorder, such as von Willebrandt's disease?
- Has anyone in the patient's family been diagnosed with a bleeding disorder?
- Has the patient ever bled excessively during surgery or, in the case of women, after giving birth?
- Does the patient have a history of easy bleeding during normal activity? For example, does the patient report bleeding for more than three minutes after brushing their teeth?
- Does the patient have physical findings suggestive of a bleeding disorder, for example, multiple bruises despite lack of significant trauma or petechia?

In the absence of any affirmative responses, perioperative coagulation screening is not recommended. In patients with a suspected bleeding disorder or a history of hypercoaguability (history of deep venous thrombosis (DVT) in the absence of trauma, history of pulmonary embolism (PE), or a family history of DVT or PE) it may be prudent to order coagulation screening and to consider an activated protein C resistance and factor V Leiden mutation test. A complete blood count (CBC) should be done in patients where there is a history of anemia, recent chemotherapy or an expected intraoperative blood loss requiring transfusion. Baseline hematocrit (HCT) testing may be warranted if surgery would be postponed in an anemic patient for iron supplementation or erythropoietin administration in anticipation of significant blood loss—eg, in a Jehovah's Witness patient.

Management of the patient with hepatic dysfunction before surgery requires identification, risk assessment, and correction of the underlying issues. While routine screening of liver function is not recommended, testing should be done for patients with suspected liver disease because of the known increased surgical morbidity and mortality.

Suspicion of hepatic dysfunction may be raised by a detailed history and physical exam. History of blood transfusions, illicit drug use, high alcohol consumption, or over-the-counter analgesics can signal liver disease. Physical signs such as temporal wasting, jaundice, spider nevi, ascites, hepatosplenomegaly, or palmar erythema may point to underlying liver pathology [8]. If liver dysfunction is suspected, serum hepatic transaminases, alkaline phosphatase, and bilirubin levels may be helpful. In extreme cases, where liver synthetic dysfunction is suspected, coagulation studies (PT and INR) should be considered.

Postoperative renal failure carries a significant mortality of 50–100% [9]. Screening for occult renal disease includes a detailed history of renal or cardiac dysfunction, vascular disease, diabetes, and hypertension. When significant renal disease is suspected or known to be present then a baseline serum creatinine, blood urea nitrogen (BUN), estimated glomerular filtration rate (GFR), comprehensive metabolic panel, and urinalysis should be considered. Patients who undergo dialysis should have electrolytes, BUN, and creatinine measured, preferably just prior to surgery to confirm safe levels before induction of anesthesia.

Summary

Laboratory evaluation of patients with spine pathology is aimed at determining underlying causes, recommending potential therapeutic options, and determining the presence of conditions that can affect surgical risk and wound healing. Preoperative screening tests are generally not warranted in otherwise healthy patients, but may be useful when the history and/or physical exam reveal the potential presence of conditions that affect perioperative risks. No single set of standard tests applies to all patients. Both general and preoperative laboratory testing are guided by the underlying cause of spinal pathology and the overall health of the patient anticipating surgical therapy. Nutritional health, particularly in patients with infection or tumor, is of paramount importance in the treatment of spinal disease and the use of correlating lab markers are advisable. Avoidance of unnecessary lab testing may be an area of substantial cost savings. Appropriate history and questionnaires may offer a more efficient use of resources.

References

1. **Stambough JL, Beringer D** (1992) Postoperative wound infections complicating adult spine surgery. *J Spinal Disord;* 5:277–285.
2. **Olsen MA, Nepple JJ, Riew KD, et al** (2008) Risk factors for surgical site infection following orthopaedic spinal operations. *J Bone Joint Surg Am;* 90:62–69.
3. **Cottle L, Riordan T** (2008) Infectious spondylodiscitis. *J Infect;* 56:401–412.
4. **Vergne P, Treves R** (1998) [Infectious spondylodiscitis. Etiology, diagnosis, progression and treatment]. *Rev Prat;* 48:2065–2071. French.
5. **Dunbar RP, Alexiades MM** (1998) Decision making in rheumatoid arthritis. Determining surgical priorities. *Rheum Dis Clin North Am;* 24:35–54.
6. **Wagner R, Jagoda A** (1997) Spinal cord syndromes. *Emerg Med Clin North Am;* 15:699–711.
7. **Bredella MA, Essary B, Torriani M, et al** (2008) Use of FDG-PET in differentiating benign from malignant compression fractures. *Skeletal Radiol;* 37:405–413.
8. **Hanje AJ, Patel T** (2007) Preoperative evaluation of patients with liver disease. *Nat Clin Pract Gastroenterol Hepatol;* 4:266–276.
9. **Novis BK, Roizen MF, Aronson S, et al** (1994) Association of preoperative risk factors with postoperative acute renal failure. *Anesth Analg;* 78:143–149.

4.1.1   Infection measurements

---

1   Blood cultures

Interpretation

Blood cultures for bacteria are positive in about 60% cases.

Why is it suitable in spine population?

Identifies organism for treatment.

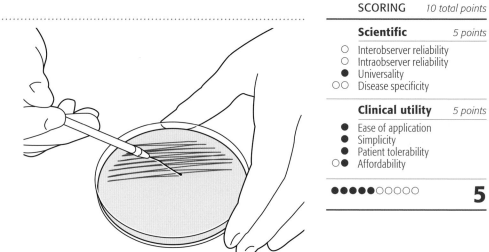

Fig 4.1.1-1

2   Tissue/bone cultures

Interpretation
Important to guide specific
antimicrobial therapy.

Why is it suitable in spine population?
Diagnosis of bacterial osteomyelitis
relies on isolation of a specific agent
from the bone or the blood.

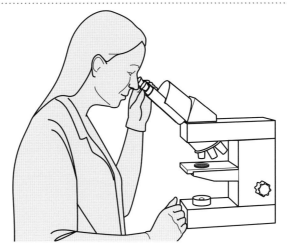

Fig 4.1.1-2

SCORING	*10 total points*

Scientific	*5 points*
○ Interobserver reliability	
○ Intraobserver reliability	
● Universality	
○○ Disease specificity	

Clinical utility	*5 points*
● Ease of application	
● Simplicity	
● Patient tolerability	
○● Affordability	

●●●●●○○○○○   **5**

3   Tuberculosis skin test

SCORING   *10 total points*

Interpretation

Routine screening outside high-risk patients leads to high false-positive test rates [1].

Why is it suitable in spine population?

Testing for latent tuberculosis infection should only be done on patients at risk of contracting M. tuberculosis or at risk of progressing from latent to active tuberculosis.

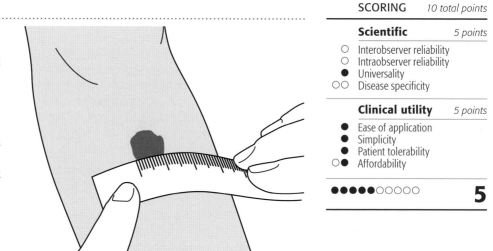

Fig 4.1.1-3

Scientific   *5 points*

○   Interobserver reliability
○   Intraobserver reliability
●   Universality
○○ Disease specificity

Clinical utility   *5 points*

●   Ease of application
●   Simplicity
●   Patient tolerability
○● Affordability

●●●●●○○○○○   **5**

References:
1. Jerant AF, Bannon M, Rittenhouse S (2000) Identification and management of tuberculosis. *Am Fam Physician;* 61(9): 2667–2678.

4   Erythrocyte sedimentation rate (ESR)

Interpretation

The test is not sensitive or specific.
There is a good correlation between
ESR and C-reactive protein as a marker
for infection.

Why is it suitable in spine population?

Nonspecific marker of infection.

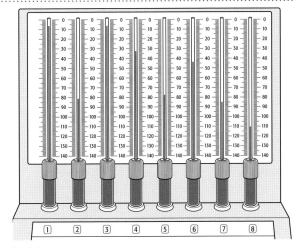

Fig 4.1.1-4

5   Complete blood count (CBC) with differential

Interpretation
Specific white cell identification
abnormality may aid in the differential
diagnosis of infectious disease
process [1].

Why is it suitable in spine
population?
CBC provides information about the
types and numbers of cells in the
blood, specifically red cells, white cells,
and platelets.

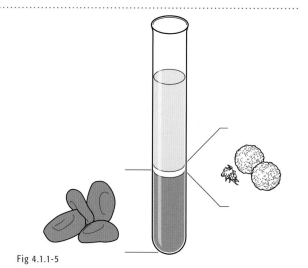

Fig 4.1.1-5

References:
1. **Gomella LG, Haist SA** (2006) Chapter 5. Laboratory Diagnosis: Clinical Hematology. *Clinician's Pocket Reference: The Scut Monkey, 11th edition.* New York: McGraw-Hill Medical, 95–108.

6   CD4 levels

Interpretation

Specific levels have been established as points for initiating prophylaxis/antiviral therapy and monitoring the efficacy of treatment. It should be monitored every 3–6 months in all HIV-infected persons [1].

Why is it suitable in spine population?

CD4 cell levels are used to help organize HIV-related clinical conditions within the Center for Disease Control's classi-fication system for HIV infection.

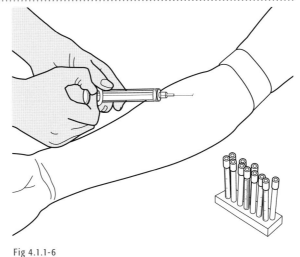

Fig 4.1.1-6

SCORING   *10 total points*

Scientific   *5 points*
○ Interobserver reliability
○ Intraobserver reliability
● Universality
○○ Disease specificity

Clinical utility   *5 points*
● Ease of application
● Simplicity
● Patient tolerability
○● Affordability

●●●●●○○○○○   **5**

References:
1. Nicoll D, McPhee SJ, Pignone M, et al (2007) *Pocket Guide to Diagnostic Tests, 5th Edition.* New York: McGraw-Hill Medical.

---

7   Human immunodeficiency virus (HIV)

Interpretation
HIV antibody test is considered positive only when a repeatedly reactive enzyme immunoassay (EIA) is confirmed by a Western blot (WB) analysis.

Why is it suitable in spine population?
This test detects antibodies against HIV-1, the etiological agent of the vast majority of all HIV infections in the USA.

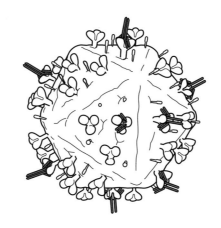

Fig 4.1.1-7

SCORING	10 total points
Scientific	5 points
○ Interobserver reliability	
○ Intraobserver reliability	
● Universality	
○○ Disease specificity	
Clinical utility	5 points
● Ease of application	
● Simplicity	
● Patient tolerability	
○● Affordability	

●●●●●○○○○○   **5**

8   Serology for suspected organisms: chlamydia, yersinia, salmonella, brucella, hydatid

Interpretation
Used to identify specific organisms.

Why is it suitable in spine population?
Used to identify specific organisms.

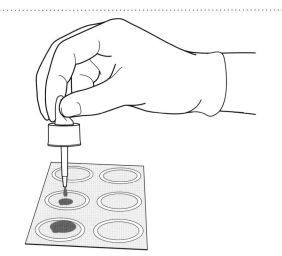

Fig 4.1.1-8

4.1.2   Rheumatological measurements

1   Serum IgA

Interpretation
Increased in systemic lupus
erythematosus (SLE), rheumatoid
arthritis, and sarcoidosis. Decreased in
nephrotic syndrome, Still disease, SLE,
common variable immunodeficiency,
and agammaglobulinemia [1].

Why is it suitable in spine population?
Can be seen as increased or decreased
depending on inflammatory or
immune disorder.

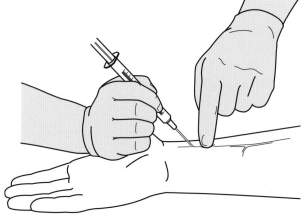

Fig 4.1.2-1

SCORING   *10 total points*

Scientific   *5 points*
- ○ Interobserver reliability
- ○ Intraobserver reliability
- ● Universality
- ○○ Disease specificity

Clinical utility   *5 points*
- ● Ease of application
- ● Simplicity
- ● Patient tolerability
- ○● Affordability

●●●●●○○○○○   **5**

References:
1. LeBlond RF, Brown DD, DeGowin RL (2008) Chapter 18. Common Laboratory Tests. *DeGowin's Diagnostic Examination, 9th Edition.* New York: McGraw-Hill Professional, 934–944.

---

2   Serum lipid levels

....

Interpretation

Decreased high-density
lipoprotein (HDL) cholesterol and
apolipoprotein A-I level, and
an increased ratio of low-density
lipoprotein (LDL) cholesterol
to HDL cholesterol levels is associated
with rheumatoid arthritis [1].

Why is it suitable in spine
population?

Elevated lipid profiles have been
identified among patients with newly
diagnosed rheumatoid arthritis.

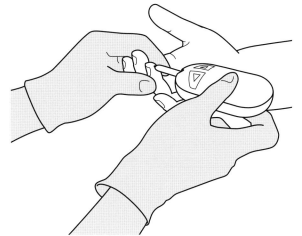

Fig 4.1.2-2

SCORING   *10 total points*

Scientific   *5 points*

○ Interobserver reliability
○ Intraobserver reliability
● Universality
○○ Disease specificity

Clinical utility   *5 points*

● Ease of application
● Simplicity
● Patient tolerability
○● Affordability

●●●●●○○○○○   **5**

References:
1. **Park YB, Lee SK, Lee WK, et al** (1999) Lipid profiles in untreated patients with rheumatoid arthritis. *J Rheumatol;* 26(8):1701–1704.

3   Rheumatoid factor

SCORING   *10 total points*

Interpretation
Due to its lack of specificity, its predictive value is low (34%) if it is used as a screening test [1, 2].

Why is it suitable in spine population?
Rheumatoid factor can be useful in differentiating rheumatoid arthritis from other chronic inflammatory arthritides. Positive in rheumatoid arthritis (75–90%).

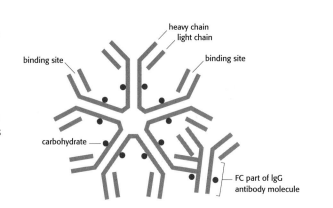

Fig 4.1.2-3

Scientific   *5 points*

○ Interobserver reliability
○ Intraobserver reliability
● Universality
○○ Disease specificity

Clinical utility   *5 points*

● Ease of application
● Simplicity
● Patient tolerability
○● Affordability

●●●●●○○○○○   **5**

References:
1. **Mierau R, Genth E** (2006) Diagnosis and prognosis of early rheumatoid arthritis, with special emphasis on laboratory analysis. *Clin Chem Lab Med;* 44(2):138–143.
2. **Westwood OM, Nelson PN, Hay FC** (2006) Rheumatoid factors: what's new? *Rheumatology (Oxford);* 45(4):379–385.

4   Antinuclear antibodies

Interpretation
Positive results can be seen in SLE, drug-induced lupus-like syndromes, scleroderma, mixed connective tissue disease, rheumatoid arthritis, polymyositis, and juvenile rheumatoid arthritis (5–20%) [1].

Why is it suitable in spine population?
Useful screening test in patients with symptoms suggesting collagen-vascular disease.

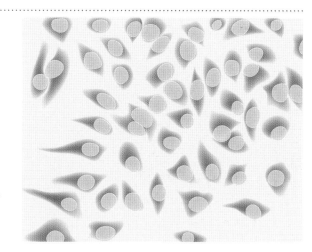

Fig 4.1.2-4

SCORING	10 total points

Scientific	5 points
○	Interobserver reliability
○	Intraobserver reliability
●	Universality
○○	Disease specificity

Clinical utility	5 points
●	Ease of application
●	Simplicity
●	Patient tolerability
○●	Affordability

●●●●●○○○○○   **5**

References:
1. **Gomella LG, Haist SA** (2006) Chapter 4. Laboratory Diagnosis: Chemistry, Immunology, Serology. *Clinician's Pocket Reference: The Scut Monkey, 11th edition.* New York: McGraw-Hill Medical, 53–94.

5   Serum amyloid A

Interpretation
Elevated levels can indicate inflammation in some autoimmune disorders such as rheumatoid arthritis and vasculitis [1].

Why is it suitable in spine population?
It is an acute-phase reactant that inceases with inflammation/disease activity.

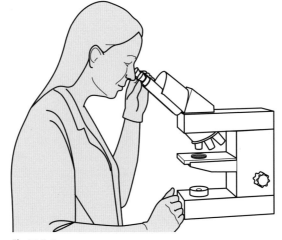

Fig 4.1.2-5

References:
1. Jovanovíc DB (2004) [Clinical importance of determination of serum amyloid A.] *Srp Arh Celok Lek;* 132(7–8):267–71. Serbian.

6   Cyclic citrullinated peptide (CCP) antibodies

Interpretation
Second-generation ELISA tests have a specificity for rheumatoid arthritis as high as 97%. Sensitivities are in the range of 70–80% for established rheumatoid arthritis and 50% for early-onset rheumatoid arthritis [1].

Why is it suitable in spine population?
Autoantibodies to citrullinated proteins are specific for rheumatoid arthritis.

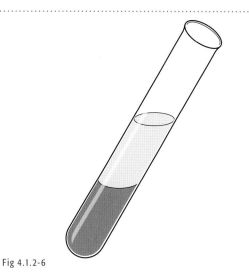

Fig 4.1.2-6

SCORING *10 total points*

Scientific *5 points*
- ○ Interobserver reliability
- ○ Intraobserver reliability
- ● Universality
- ○○ Disease specificity

Clinical utility *5 points*
- ● Ease of application
- ● Simplicity
- ● Patient tolerability
- ○● Affordability

●●●●●○○○○○   **5**

References:
1. **Imboden JB** (2006) Chapter 3. Laboratory Diagnosis. *Imboden JB, Hellmann DB, Stone JH (eds), CURRENT Diagnosis & Treatment in Rheumatology, 2nd edition.* New York: McGraw-Hill Professional.

7   HLA-B27

SCORING   *10 total points*

Interpretation

Positive in 88% of patients with ankylosing spondylitis. It is also associated with the development of Reiter syndrome (80%) following infection with enteric organisms, such as yersinia, shigella, or salmonella [1].

Why is it suitable in spine population?

Positive in patients with spondyloarthritis and Reiter syndrome.

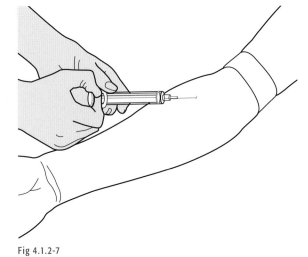

Fig 4.1.2-7

Scientific   *5 points*

○ Interobserver reliability
○ Intraobserver reliability
● Universality
○○ Disease specificity

Clinical utility   *5 points*

● Ease of application
● Simplicity
● Patient tolerability
○● Affordability

●●●●●○○○○○   **5**

References:
1. Nicoll D, McPhee SJ, Pignone M, et al (2007) *Pocket Guide to Diagnostic Tests, 5th Edition.* New York: McGraw-Hill Medical.

4.1.3   Clotting function measurements

---

1   Prothrombin time (PT)/international normalized ratio (INR)

Interpretation
Bleeding is increased three-fold in patients with INRs of 3.0–4.5 than in patients with INRs of 2.0–3.0 [1].

Why is it suitable in spine population?
Looks at the different coagulation pathways.

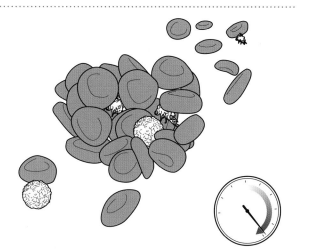

SCORING   *10 total points*

Scientific	*5 points*
○ Interobserver reliability	
○ Intraobserver reliability	
● Universality	
○○ Disease specificity	

Clinical utility	*5 points*
● Ease of application	
● Simplicity	
● Patient tolerability	
○● Affordability	

●●●●●○○○○○   **5**

Normal reference range

INR

Female		Male	
Age (years)	Range (U/L)	Age (years)	Range (U/L)
0–	0.8–1.3	0–	0.8–1.3

PT

Female		Male	
Age (years)	Range (U/L)	Age (years)	Range (U/L)
0–	10.7–15.6	0–	10.7–15.6

Fig 4.1.3-1

References:
1. Nicoll D, McPhee SJ, Pignone M, et al (2007) *Pocket Guide to Diagnostic Tests, 5th Edition.* New York: McGraw-Hill Medical.

2   Partial thromboplastin time (PTT)

Interpretation
Used to evaluate clotting ability.

Why is it suitable in spine population?
Considers the different coagulation pathways and coagulation factors except XIII and VII.

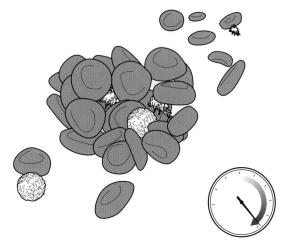

Normal reference range

PTT

Female		Male	
Age (years)	Range (U/L)	Age (years)	Range (U/L)
0–	22–35	0–	22–35

Fig 4.1.3-2

3   Platelet function

Interpretation
Normal PFA-100 CT excludes some
severe platelet defects, however not as
accurate for mild platelet disorders.

Why is it suitable in spine population?
Measures platelet adhesion and
aggregation.

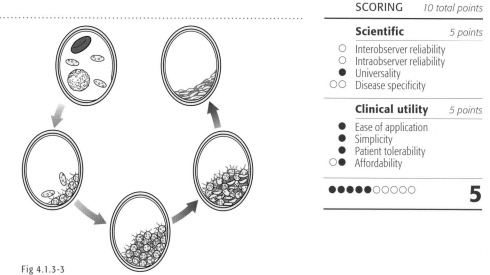

Fig 4.1.3-3

SCORING   *10 total points*

Scientific   *5 points*
○ Interobserver reliability
○ Intraobserver reliability
● Universality
○○ Disease specificity

Clinical utility   *5 points*
● Ease of application
● Simplicity
● Patient tolerability
○● Affordability

●●●●●○○○○○   **5**

---

4   **Fibrinogen**

....

Interpretation
An assay is done to investigate unexplained bleeding, prolonged PT or PTT, or as part of a disseminated intravascular coagulation panel.

Why is it suitable in spine population?
It is cleaved by thrombin forming insoluble fibrin monomers that polymerize to make a clot.

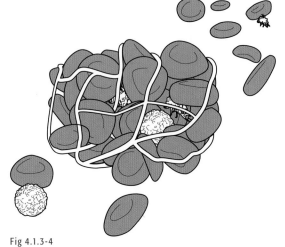

Fig 4.1.3-4

5   Activated protein C resistance (APCR)

Interpretation
Patients with APCR are more likely to have deep and superficial venous thromboses. Less commonly seen are primary pulmonary embolisms [1].

Why is it suitable in spine population?
Resistance of plasma to the anticoagulant effects of activated protein C.

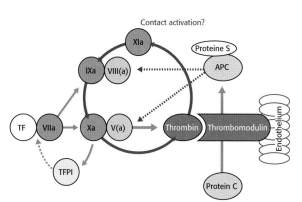

Fig 4.1.3-5

References:
1. **Seligsohn U, Griffin JH** (2008) Chapter 122. Hereditary Thrombophilia. *Lichtman M, Beutler E, Kipps TJ, Kaushansky K (eds), Williams Hematology, 7th Edition.* New York: McGraw-Hill Professional, 1981–2008.

6   Factor V Leiden mutation test

SCORING   *10 total points*

Interpretation

This would indicate a risk factor for thrombosis.

Why is it suitable in spine population?

This mutation results in a significantly reduced anticoagulant response to activated protein C.

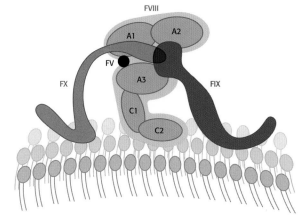

Fig 4.1.3-6

Scientific   *5 points*

○ Interobserver reliability
○ Intraobserver reliability
● Universality
○○ Disease specificity

Clinical utility   *5 points*

● Ease of application
● Simplicity
● Patient tolerability
○● Affordability

●●●●●○○○○○   **5**

4.1.4   Hepatorenal function measurements

1   Alanine aminotransferase (ALAT)

Interpretation
ALAT is the preferred enzyme for evaluation of liver injury in high-risk populations.

Why is it suitable in spine population?
Intracellular enzyme involved in amino acid metabolism.

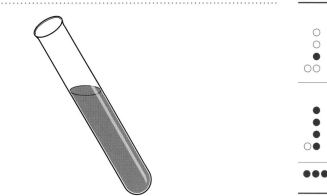

Normal reference range

Female		Male	
Age (years)	Range (U/L)	Age (years)	Range (U/L)
0–	6–40	0–49	10–64
		50	10–48

Fig 4.1.4-1

SCORING   *10 total points*

Scientific   *5 points*
○   Interobserver reliability
○   Intraobserver reliability
●   Universality
○○ Disease specificity

Clinical utility   *5 points*
●   Ease of application
●   Simplicity
●   Patient tolerability
○● Affordability

●●●●●○○○○○   **5**

2   Aspartate aminotransferase (ASAT)

Interpretation
Increased in:
- Acute viral hepatitis (ALT > AST)
- Biliary tract obstruction
- Alcohol-induced hepatitis and cirrhosis (AST > ALT)
- Liver abscess
- Metastatic or primary liver cancer
- Right heart failure
- Ischemia or hypoxia
- Injury to the liver
- Extensive trauma

Why is it suitable in spine population?
Intracellular enzyme involved in amino acid metabolism. Released into the bloodstream when liver tissue is damaged.

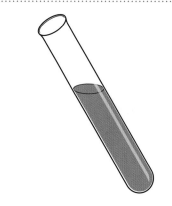

Normal reference range

Female		Male	
Age (years)	Range (U/L)	Age (years)	Range (U/L)
0–	15–40	0–	15–40

Fig 4.1.4-2

SCORING   *10 total points*

Scientific   *5 points*
- ○ Interobserver reliability
- ○ Intraobserver reliability
- ● Universality
- ○○ Disease specificity

Clinical utility   *5 points*
- ● Ease of application
- ● Simplicity
- ● Patient tolerability
- ○● Affordability

●●●●●○○○○○   **5**

---

3   Alkaline phosphatase (AFOS)

Interpretation
Used to measure the extent of bone metastases in prostate cancer.

Why is it suitable in spine population?
Alkaline phosphatases are found in the liver, bone, intestine, and placenta.

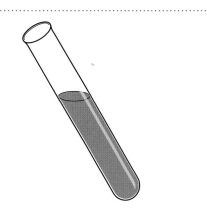

Normal reference range

Female		Male	
Age (years)	Range (U/L)	Age (years)	Range (U/L)
0–9	111–281	0–9	115–324
10–11	132–366	10–11	115–324
12–13	89–285	12–13	119–426
14–17	43–226	14–17	72–400
18–24	26–98	18–24	42–136
25–34	25–100	25–34	35–109
35–44	25–112	35–44	36–122
45–54	34–121	45–54	39–139
55–64	31–132	55–64	37–159
65–74	38–172	65–74	36–161
75–	49–199	75–	52–227

Fig 4.1.4-3

4   Bilirubin—total and direct

SCORING   *10 total points*

Scientific   *5 points*

○ Interobserver reliability
○ Intraobserver reliability
● Universality
○○ Disease specificity

Clinical utility   *5 points*

● Ease of application
● Simplicity
● Patient tolerability
○● Affordability

●●●●●○○○○○   **5**

Interpretation
Elevated serum bilirubin occurs in liver disease, biliary obstruction, or hemolysis.

Why is it suitable in spine population?
A product of hemoglobin metabolism.

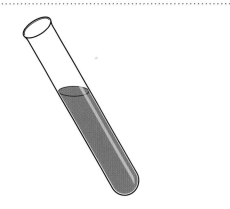

Normal reference range

Direct

Female		Male	
Age (years)	Range (mg/dL)	Age (years)	Range (mg/dL)
0–	0.0–0.3	0–	0.0–0.3

Total

Female		Male	
Age (months)	Range (mg/dL)	Age (months)	Range (mg/dL)
0–0	0.2–1.3	0–0	0.2–1.3
1	0.2–1.3	1	0.2–1.3

Fig 4.1.4-4

---

5   Serum albumin

....

Interpretation
Low serum albumin indicates severity in chronic liver disease.

Why is it suitable in spine population?
Major component of plasma proteins. Affected by nutritional state, hepatic and renal function, and various other diseases.

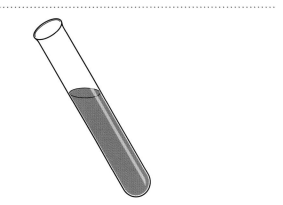

Normal reference range

Female		Male	
Age (years)	Range (g/dL)	Age (years)	Range (g/dL)
0–	3.5–5.2	0–	3.5–5.2

Fig 4.1.4-5

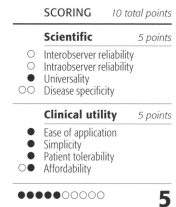

SCORING   *10 total points*

Scientific   *5 points*
○ Interobserver reliability
○ Intraobserver reliability
● Universality
○○ Disease specificity

Clinical utility   *5 points*
● Ease of application
● Simplicity
● Patient tolerability
○● Affordability

●●●●●○○○○○   **5**

6   Total protein

Interpretation

Increased alpha 2 indicates nephrotic syndrome, inflammatory states.

Decreased alpha 2 in vivo indicates hemolysis and liver disease [1].

Why is it suitable in spine population?

Separates albumin into different fractions that in different ratios can indicate hepatorenal disease states.

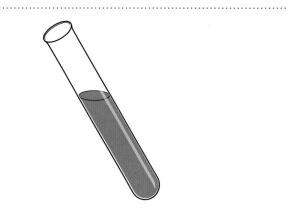

Normal reference range

Female		Male	
Age (years)	Range (g/dL)	Age (years)	Range (g/dL)
0–	6.0–8.2	0–	6.0–8.2

Fig 4.1.4-6

References:
1. Nicoll D, McPhee SJ, Pignone M, et al (2007) *Pocket Guide to Diagnostic Tests, 5th Edition.* New York: McGraw-Hill Medical.

7   Creatine kinase total activity

Interpretation

Increased level is associated with marked damage to nephrons, making the test not a good indicator of early disease.

Why is it suitable in spine population?

Evaluates renal function.

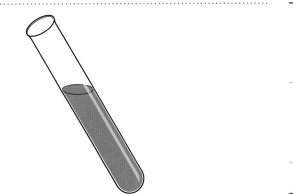

Normal reference range

Female		Male	
Age (years)	Range (U/L)	Age (years)	Range (U/L)
0–	30–231	0–	30–285

Fig 4.1.4-7

8   Blood urea nitrogen (BUN)

Interpretation
Elevated with renal or urinary tract obstruction or dehydration. It will be reduced in hepatic failure, nephrotic syndrome, or in cachectic patients.

Why is it suitable in spine population?
Can further elucidate hepatorenal failure.

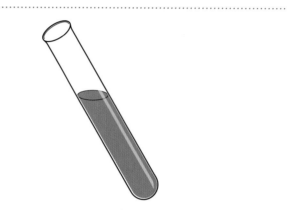

Normal reference range

Female		Male	
Age (years)	Range (mg/dL)	Age (years)	Range (mg/dL)
0–	8–21	0–	8–21

Fig 4.1.4-8

SCORING   *10 total points*

Scientific   *5 points*
- ○ Interobserver reliability
- ○ Intraobserver reliability
- ● Universality
- ○○ Disease specificity

Clinical utility   *5 points*
- ● Ease of application
- ● Simplicity
- ● Patient tolerability
- ○● Affordability

●●●●●○○○○○   **5**

9   Estimated glomerular filtration rate (EGFR)

Interpretation
Renal failure is defined as glomerular filtration rate (GFR) <15 mL/min.

GFR is calculated by the Modification of Diet in Renal Disease (MDRD) Study equation, which is reasonably accurate in non-hospitalized patients with chronic kidney disease, but tends to underestimate GFR in other populations.
It is inaccurate in patients with rapidly changing renal function [1].

Why is it suitable in spine population?
Equation to quantify renal damage.

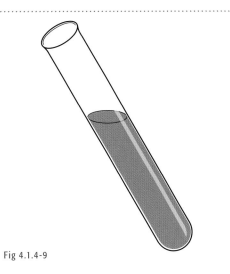

Fig 4.1.4-9

SCORING   *10 total points*

Scientific   *5 points*
○ Interobserver reliability
○ Intraobserver reliability
● Universality
○○ Disease specificity

Clinical utility   *5 points*
● Ease of application
● Simplicity
● Patient tolerability
○● Affordability

●●●●●○○○○○   **5**

References:
1. Stevens LA, Coresh J, Greene T, et al (2006) Assessing kidney function—measured and estimated glomerular filtration rate. *N Engl J Med;* 354:2473–2483.

4.1.5   Comprehensive metabolic panel

1   Urinalysis

Interpretation
Useful in identifying some renal
tubular dysfunction and nonrenal
disturbances [1].

Why is it suitable in spine population?
Simple test to evaluate renal function.

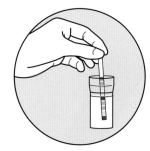
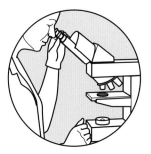

Fig 4.1.5-1

SCORING   *10 total points*

Scientific   *5 points*
○ Interobserver reliability
○ Intraobserver reliability
● Universality
○○ Disease specificity

Clinical utility   *5 points*
● Ease of application
● Simplicity
● Patient tolerability
○● Affordability

●●●●●○○○○○   **5**

References:
1. Morgan GE Jr, Mikhail MS, Murray MJ (2005) Chapter 32. Anesthesia for Patients with renal disease. *Clinical Anesthesiology, 4th edition.* New York: McGraw-Hill Medical, 742–756.

4.1.6   Bone mineral metabolism

---

1   Parathyroid hormone levels

....

Interpretation
Increased in vitamin D deficiency.

Why is it suitable in spine population?
Evaluates potential vitamin D system function.

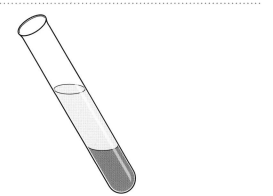

Normal reference range

Female		Male	
Age (years)	Range (pg/mL)	Age (years)	Range (pg/mL)
0–	12–88	0–	12–88

Fig 4.1.6-1

2   Serum calcium: total, free, ionized

Interpretation

Decreased in renal insufficiency, excessive fluid intake, malabsorption of calcium and vitamin D or dietary vitamin D deficiency (osteomalacia and rickets), hypoproteinemia (cachexia, nephrosis, celiac disease, cystic fibrosis of the pancreas), certain drugs (antacids), corticosteroids. Vitamin D deficiency or impaired metabolism.

Increased vitamin D intoxication, milk-alkali syndrome, hyperproteinemia (sarcoidosis, multiple myeloma) [1].

Why is it suitable in spine population?

Vitamin D intoxication, milk-alkali syndrome, and hyperproteinemia (sarcoidosis, multiple myeloma).

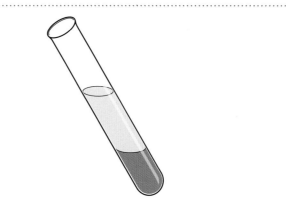

Normal reference range

Female		Male	
Age (years)	Range (mg/dL)	Age (years)	Range (mg/dL)
0–	8.9–10.2	0–	8.9–10.2

Fig 4.1.6-2

SCORING   *10 total points*

Scientific   *5 points*
○ Interobserver reliability
○ Intraobserver reliability
● Universality
○○ Disease specificity

Clinical utility   *5 points*
● Ease of application
● Simplicity
● Patient tolerability
○● Affordability

●●●●●○○○○○   **5**

References:
1. LeBlond RF, Brown DD, DeGowin RL (2008) Chapter 18. Common Laboratory Tests. *DeGowin's Diagnostic Examination, 9th Edition.* New York: McGraw-Hill Professional, 934–944.

3   Phosphate: serum and urine

Interpretation

Decreased with impaired absorption (diarrhea, vitamin D deficiency, impaired metabolism).

Increased exogenous phosphorus load or absorption, phosphorus-containing laxatives or enemas, vitamin D excess [1].

Why is it suitable in spine population?

Serum phosphate is a poor reflection of body stores because <1% of the phosphate is in extracellular fluid.

Bones serve as a reservoir. However still useful in defining nutrition status.

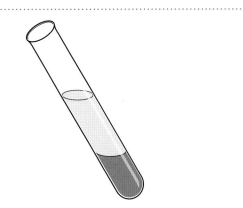

Normal reference range

Female		Male	
Age (years)	Range (mg/dL)	Age (years)	Range (mg/dL)
0–11	4.5–6.0	0–11	4.5–6.0
12–	2.4–4.5	12–	2.4–4.5

Fig 4.1.6-3

References:
1. **Charney P, Malone A** (2004) *ADA Pocket Guide to Nutrition Assessment.* Chicago: Amer Dietetic Assn.

4   Alkaline phosphate/serum bone–specific alkaline phosphatase

SCORING   *10 total points*

Interpretation
Increased in osteoblastic bone tumors (metastatic or osteogenic sarcoma), osteomalacia, and rickets.

Decreased in malnutrition, excess vitamin D ingestion, pernicious anemia, Wilson disease, hypothyroidism, and zinc deficiency [1].

Why is it suitable in spine population?
Normal serum alkaline phosphatase consists of many distinct isoenzymes found in the liver, bone, placenta, and, less commonly, small intestine.

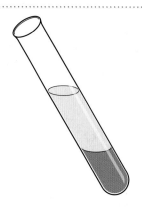

Scientific   *5 points*
- ○ Interobserver reliability
- ○ Intraobserver reliability
- ● Universality
- ○○ Disease specificity

Clinical utility   *5 points*
- ● Ease of application
- ● Simplicity
- ● Patient tolerability
- ○● Affordability

●●●●●○○○○○   **5**

Normal reference range

Age (years)	Range (µg/L)
18–29	8.4–29.3
30–39	7.7–21.3
40–49	7.0–18.3
50–68	7.6–14.9

≥ 18 year old females:

Age (years)	Range (µg/L)
18–29	4.7–17.8
30–39	5.3–19.5
40–49	5.0–18.8
50–76	5.6–29.0

Premenopausal (35–45 years)

Fig 4.1.6-4

References:
1. **Gomella LG, Haist SA** (2006) Chapter 4. Laboratory Diagnosis: Chemistry, Immunology, Serology. *Clinician's Pocket Reference: The Scut Monkey, 11th edition.* New York: McGraw-Hill Medical, 53–94.

5   Tubular reabsorption of phosphate

Interpretation
Can be associated with dysfunctional proximal tubular function of the renal tract, such as Fanconi syndrome [1].

Why is it suitable in spine population?
Evaluates for renal phosphate wasting.

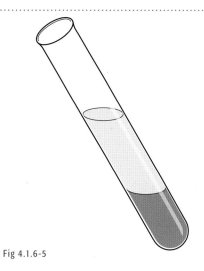

Fig 4.1.6-5

References:
1. **Salant DJ, Patel PS,** Chapter 278. Polycystic Kidney Disease and Other Inherited Tubular Disorders. *Fauci AS, Braunwald E, Kasper DL, et al (eds), Harrison's Principles of Internal Medicine, 17th edition.* New York: McGraw-Hill Professional.

6   Urine cyclic AMP

SCORING   *10 total points*

Interpretation
High urinary cyclic adenosine monophosphate excretion suggests lack of vitamin D and secondary hyperparathyroidism [1].

Why is it suitable in spine population?
Used to evaluate vitamin D deficiency.

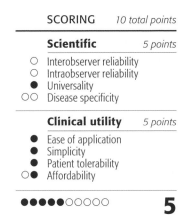

Scientific   *5 points*

○ Interobserver reliability
○ Intraobserver reliability
● Universality
○○ Disease specificity

Clinical utility   *5 points*

● Ease of application
● Simplicity
● Patient tolerability
○● Affordability

●●●●●○○○○○   **5**

Normal reference range

Glomerular filtrate	1.3–3.7 (nmol/dL)

Fig 4.1.6-6

References:
1. von Lilienfeld-Toal H, Mackes KG, Kodrat G, et al (1977) Plasma 25-hydroxyvitamin D and urinary cyclic AMP in German patients with subtotal gastrectomy (Billroth II). *Am J Dig Dis;* 22(7):633–666.

7   Serum vitamin D (25-hydroxyvitamin D) levels

Interpretation

Measurement of serum vitamin D indicates both vitamin D deficiency and toxicity. Useful for hypocalcemic disorders related to increased PTH levels, and in patients with rickets and osteomalacia [1].

Why is it suitable in spine population?

Evaluates the ability of the vitamin D system to maintain serum calcium levels.

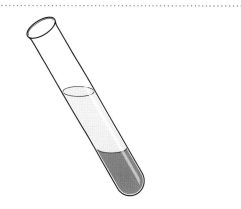

Scientific   *5 points*

○   Interobserver reliability
○   Intraobserver reliability
●   Universality
○○ Disease specificity

Clinical utility   *5 points*

●   Ease of application
●   Simplicity
●   Patient tolerability
○● Affordability

●●●●●○○○○○   **5**

Normal reference range

Total

Female		Male	
Age (years)	Range (ng/mL)	Age (years)	Range (ng/mL)
0–	20.1–50.0	0–	20.1–50.0

Fig 4.1.6-7

References:
1. Nicoll D, McPhee SJ, Pignone M, et al (2007) *Pocket Guide to Diagnostic Tests, 5th Edition.* New York: McGraw-Hill Medical.

8   Thyroid function studies: thyroid-stimulating hormone (TSH), T3, free T4

Interpretation

Serum TSH is ordered to evaluate basic hypothyroidism and hyperthyroidism. When suspicion is moderate to high both the serum TSH and free T4 should be ordered. If thyroid dysfunction is clinically obvious or confirmed, then serum T3 is useful to identify the cause and plan the therapy [1].

Why is it suitable in spine population?

Evaluation of thyroid dysfunction and neoplasia.

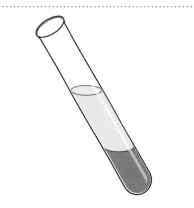

Normal reference range

TSH

Female		Male	
Age (years)	Range (uiU/mL)	Age (years)	Range (uiU/mL)
0–	0.400–5.000	0–	0.400–5.000

T3

Female		Male	
Age (years)	Range (mcg/dL)	Age (years)	Range (mcg/dL)
0–	73–178	0–	73–178

T4

Female		Male	
Age (months)	Range (mcg/dL)	Age (months)	Range (mcg/dL)
0–	4.8–10.8	0–	4.8–10.8
1–	4.8–10.8	1–	4.8–10.8

Fig 4.1.6-8

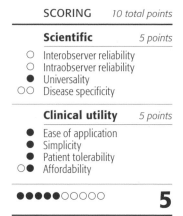

SCORING   *10 total points*

Scientific   *5 points*

○ Interobserver reliability
○ Intraobserver reliability
● Universality
○○ Disease specificity

Clinical utility   *5 points*

● Ease of application
● Simplicity
● Patient tolerability
○● Affordability

●●●●●○○○○○   **5**

References:
1. Cooper DS, Greenspan FS, Ladenson PW (2007) The Thyroid Gland. *Gardner DG, Shoback D (eds), Greenspan's Basic and Clinical Endocrinology, 8th Edition.* New York: McGraw-Hill Medical, 209.

9   Serum vitamin B12 levels

Interpretation

Decreased levels in pernicious anemia, gastrectomy, gastric carcinoma, and malabsorptive states [1].

Why is it suitable in spine population?

Work up of certain anemia and malabsorptive states.

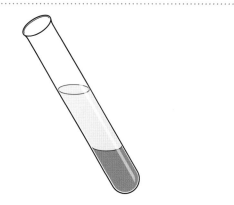

Normal reference range

Female		Male	
Age (years)	Range (pg/mL)	Age (years)	Range (pg/mL)
0–	180–914	0–	180–914

Fig 4.1.6-9

SCORING   *10 total points*

Scientific   *5 points*
- ○ Interobserver reliability
- ○ Intraobserver reliability
- ● Universality
- ○○ Disease specificity

Clinical utility   *5 points*
- ● Ease of application
- ● Simplicity
- ● Patient tolerability
- ○● Affordability

●●●●●○○○○○   **5**

References:
1. Nicoll D, McPhee SJ, Pignone M, et al (2007) *Pocket Guide to Diagnostic Tests, 5th Edition.* New York: McGraw-Hill Medical.

10   Amino-terminal propeptide of type 1 procollagen

Interpretation
In known cancer it is used to predict
bone metastases, disease progression,
and survival [1, 2].

Why is it suitable in spine population?
A new marker of bone formation.

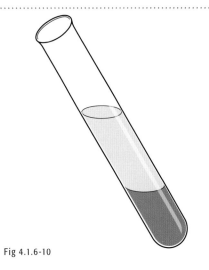

Fig 4.1.6-10

References:
1. **Thurairaja R, Iles RK, Jefferson K, et al** (2006) Serum amino-terminal propeptide of type 1 procollagen (P1NP) in prostate cancer: a potential predictor of bone metastases and prognosticator for disease progression and survival. *Urol Int;* 76(1):67–71.
2. **Oremek G, Sauer-Eppel H, Klepzig M** (2007) Total procollagen type 1 amino-terminal propeptide (total P1NP) as a bone metastasis marker in gynecological carcinomas. *Anticancer Res;* 27(4A):1961–1962.

11   Urine bone markers (N-telopeptide)

Interpretation
Monitors bone metabolism by looking at end products of bone [1].

Scientific   *5 points*

○ Interobserver reliability
○ Intraobserver reliability
● Universality
○○ Disease specificity

Why is it suitable in spine population?
Biochemical marker of human bone resorption.

Clinical utility   *5 points*

● Ease of application
● Simplicity
● Patient tolerability
○● Affordability

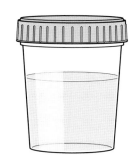

●●●●●○○○○○   **5**

Normal reference range

Adult males	21–83 nM BCE/mM Creat
Premenopausal adult females	17–94 nM BCE/mM Creat
Postmenopausal adult females	26–124 nM BCE/mM Creat

Fig 4.1.6-11

References:
1. **Gomella LG, Haist SA** (2006) Chapter 4. *Laboratory Diagnosis: Chemistry, Immunology, Serology. Clinician's Pocket Reference: The Scut Monkey, 11th edition.* New York: McGraw-Hill Medical, 53–94.

12   Serum telopeptides

Interpretation
Monitors bone metabolism, if the use
of urine is not possible.

Why is it suitable in spine population?
Biochemical marker of human bone
resorption.

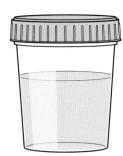

Normal reference range

Adult males	5.4–24.2 nM BCE
Premenopausal adult females	6.2–19.0 nM BCE

Fig 4.1.6-12

SCORING   *10 total points*

Scientific   *5 points*
○ Interobserver reliability
○ Intraobserver reliability
● Universality
○○ Disease specificity

Clinical utility   *5 points*
● Ease of application
● Simplicity
● Patient tolerability
○● Affordability

●●●●●○○○○○   **5**

13   Urine hydroxyproline

Interpretation
Nonspecific marker for bone resorption
but it lacks sensitivity and specificity [1].

Why is it suitable in spine population?
Biochemical marker of human bone
resorption.

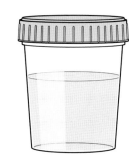

Normal reference range

Free	0–30 umol/24 hours
Total	38–500 umol/24 hours

Fig 4.1.6-13

SCORING   *10 total points*

Scientific   *5 points*
○ Interobserver reliability
○ Intraobserver reliability
● Universality
○○ Disease specificity

Clinical utility   *5 points*
● Ease of application
● Simplicity
● Patient tolerability
○● Affordability

●●●●●○○○○○   **5**

References:
1. Simsek B, Karacaer O, Karaca I (2004) Urine products of bone breakdown as markers of bone resorption and clinical usefulness of urinary hydroxyproline: an overview. *Chin Med J (Engl)*; 117(2):291–295.

4.1.7   Toxicology screens

1   Serum toxicology screen

Interpretation
These panels are institutionally variable. There is an array of values depending on the substance in question.

Why is it suitable in spine population?
Indicative of consumption of substances, both legal and illegal, which may reflect patient compliance and behaviour.

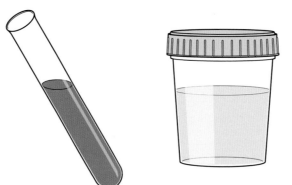

Fig 4.1.7-1

SCORING   *10 total points*

Scientific   *5 points*
○ Interobserver reliability
○ Intraobserver reliability
● Universality
○○ Disease specificity

Clinical utility   *5 points*
● Ease of application
● Simplicity
● Patient tolerability
○● Affordability

●●●●●○○○○○   **5**

2   Serum ferritin

Interpretation
Seen in blood lead concentrations higher than mcg/dL [1].

Why is it suitable in spine population?
Evaluates blood lead concentrations— as work up of peripheral neuropathy (painless weakness of the extensors resulting in classic wrist-drop).

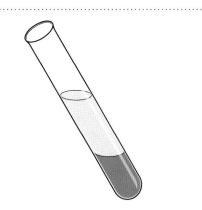

Normal reference range

Age	Range (ng/mL)	Range (mcg/L)
Newborns	25–200	25–200 [2]
Children (1 month)	200–600	200–600 [2]
Children (2–5months)	50–200	50–200 [2]
Children (6 months–15 years)	7–140	7–140 [2]
Adult males	30–300	30–300 [3]
Adult females	10–200	10–200 [3]

Fig 4.1.7-2

References:
1. **Kosnett MJ** (2009) Heavy Metal Intoxication & Chelators. *Katzung BG, Masters S, Trevor A (eds), Basic and Clinical Pharmacology, 11th edition.* New York: Mc Graw-Hill Medical.
2. **Tietz NW** (1995): Clinical Guide to Laboratory Tests, 3rd ed. *Philadelphia, PA, W. B. Saunders.*
3. **Kratz A, Ferraro M, Sluss PM, et al** (2004): Case records of the Massachusetts General Hospital: laboratory values. *N Engl J Med;* 351(15):1549-1563.

---

3   Serum aluminum

Interpretation
May develop osteomalacia due to excess aluminum. From aluminum-containing antacids or long-term total parenteral nutrition [1].

Why is it suitable in spine population?
Evaluation of bone mineralization inhibition.

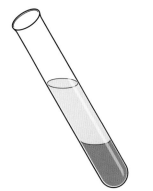

Normal reference range

Age (years)	Range (ng/mL)
All ages	0–6
Dialysis patients all ages	<60

Fig 4.1.7-3

SCORING   *10 total points*

Scientific   *5 points*
○ Interobserver reliability
○ Intraobserver reliability
● Universality
○○ Disease specificity

Clinical utility   *5 points*
● Ease of application
● Simplicity
● Patient tolerability
○● Affordability

●●●●●○○○○○   **5**

References:
1. **Fitzgerald PA** (2009) Endocrine Disorders. *McPhee SJ, Papadakis MA (eds), CURRENT Medical Diagnosis & Treatment 2010, 49th Edition.* New York: McGraw-Hill Medical.

4.1.8   Oncologic bone disease

---

1   Serum protein electrophoresis

....

Interpretation
Elevated alpha-2 globulins gamma
zones are associated malignancies [1].

**Why is it suitable in spine
population?**
Analysis of serum proteins as work-up
of hypoglobulinemia, macroglobulinemia, 1-antitrypsin deficiency,
collagen disease, liver disease, and
myeloma.

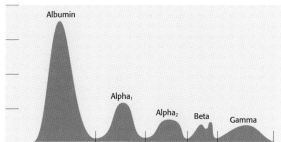

Fig 4.1.8-1

References:
1. Nicoll D, McPhee SJ, Pignone M, et al (2007) *Pocket Guide to Diagnostic Tests, 5th Edition.* New York: McGraw-Hill Medical.

2   Urine protein electrophoresis

....

Interpretation
Associated with myeloma,
Waldenström macroglobulinemia,
and Fanconi syndrome [1].

Why is it suitable in spine population?
Used to detect Bence Jones protein.

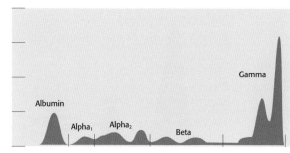

Fig 4.1.8-2

References:
1. Gomella LG, Haist SA (2006) Chapter 4. Laboratory Diagnosis: Chemistry, Immunology, Serology. *Clinician's Pocket Reference: The Scut Monkey, 11th edition.* New York: McGraw-Hill Medical, 53–94.

4   Laboratory measurements
4.2   Electrophysiological measurements

4   Laboratory measurements

4.2   Electrophysiological measurements

Introduction

Electrophysiological monitoring refers to a set of techniques that are utilized in both clinical outpatient settings and in surgery to assess the health and function of a patient's nervous system. Their use in evaluating nervous system function goes back to the early 20th century, when such techniques were used to locate epileptic foci during surgery as well as to aid in the localization of the facial nerve during acoustic neuroma surgeries [1, 2]. Eventually such techniques were adapted to surgeries involving the spinal cord in an effort to protect the spinal cord from injury during surgeries requiring severe spine correction, such as scoliosis surgery [3–5]. Other uses have evolved as well, both in clinical settings and in surgery, and are now viewed as a standard of care in most spine care settings in the USA [6, 7].

Purpose

Electrophysiological monitoring of spinal cord function can be broadly divided into two categories—intraoperative monitoring and outpatient clinical tests. Each serves a distinct purpose, but in the end, each application provides a relatively direct assessment of the condition of the spinal cord and the associated spinal nerve roots.

Intraoperative neurophysiological monitoring (IONM) is a form of electrophysiological monitoring where specific electrophysiological tests are applied to a patient's nervous system during surgery in order to evaluate its function. Historically, such testing was initially done only during severe spine correction surgeries such as scoliosis and kyphosis, when both the spinal cord and its blood supply were put in serious risk following a correction in spinal alignment. However, as the number and types of spine procedures has grown over the last 25 years, the demand for neuroprotection during spine surgeries has increased. Consequently, IONM has evolved to provide a more complete picture of spine health. It is routinely used to evaluate sensory and motor function of the spinal cord as well as to monitor the condition of spinal cord motor nerve roots during surgery. Presently at many institutions, IONM is the standard of care and used during nearly all spine procedures that involve instrumentation, as well as many others that place the spinal cord or spinal nerve roots in harm's way.

Electrophysiological monitoring in the clinic serves a different but related goal: identification and localization of neurological abnormalities. Frequently, such testing is used following or as an addendum to a more traditional physical examination when a neurological deficit is noted. The testing provides a more direct, standardized measure of the deficit as well as a mechanism to localize the neurological abnormality. Most institutions in the USA routinely use clinical electrophysiological tests.

Relevance

Electrophysiological evaluation of spinal cord function in the operating room, or in the clinical setting, involves the administration of a set of tests to the subject's nervous system, and the subsequent evaluation of the results of these tests. The interpretation and evaluation will depend on the purpose of the test. In the operating room, the purpose of testing is to protect the patient's nervous system against injury as a result of the surgical procedure. Thus results during the procedure are generally interpreted against a control set of results obtained from the patient prior to the surgical procedure. In some instances, however, a set of standard expected results will be used to evaluate preoperative pathologies intraoperatively. In the clinic, the goal of electrophysiological testing is quite different. Results of electrophysiological testing will be typically compared against a standard patient population in an effort to diagnose, evaluate, and localize any neuropathologies in a patient.

Electrophysiological testing in spine care can be generally divided into two broad categories: evaluation of sensory function and evaluation of motor function. Examination of sensory function generally utilizes somatosensory evoked potentials (SEP), dermatomal somatosensory evoked potentials (dSEP), and H-reflexes. Such testing can be used to evaluate overall spinal cord health, sensory nerve root health, and peripheral nerve and nerve root pathologies. Testing of a patient's motor function typically involves the use of transcranial motor evoked potentials (tcMEP, or MEP) as well as electromyography (EMG). Each of the above tests can be used to evaluate different aspects of a patient's nervous system, and can be applied differently, depending upon the goal of the study.

Sensory evoked potentials (SEP)
SEPs and dSEPs are tests that are used to assess the integrity and condition of the sensory nervous system of a patient. SEPs

are frequently applied to a patient in the operating room to assess intraoperatively the condition of a patient's spinal cord. Use of SEPs has been reported to improve outcome in high-risk spine procedures, such as scoliosis correction surgeries [8]. Their usefulness for the numerous other types of invasive spine procedures is presumed, but as yet not clearly demonstrated in the literature, due to the difficulty of performing randomized controlled studies using the technique. Nevertheless, SEPs are routinely used in the operating room and are considered the standard of care at most institutions.

SEPs can also be used in the clinic to assess a patient's spinal cord function, and have been used to diagnose lumbar spine stenosis and radiculopathies [9–12]. In addition, dSEPs can also be used in the clinic to diagnose specific spinal nerve root radiculopathies as well as spinal stenosis. With dSEPs, specific areas of the skin are stimulated, in order to assess transmission through the nerve roots serving that area. A reduction in signal indicates nerve root compression [13–16]. However, there is some controversy regarding the specificity and utility of dSEPs in the diagnosis of radiculopathies [17–21]. dSEPs could provide valuable information in the operating room as well. However, they are technically demanding in the operating room setting, and may be unreliable due to their high sensitivity to local and volatile anesthetic agents [22–25].

One final application of SEPs is H-wave testing. The H-wave is a basic spinal cord reflex that involves single-level sensory nerve fibers and roots along with the complimentary motor nerve roots and fibers. H-waves are stimulated bilaterally, and then the results are compared. Typically, H-wave testing is used to diagnose S1 nerve root disorders, and unlike EMG, can detect sensory lesions, along with proximal and compressive ones [10, 26–29]. However, a normal H-wave may be observed even in the presence of a radiculopathy [9], and any peripheral neuropathies need to be ruled out. In the operating room, H-wave testing has been shown to be a sensitive detector of acute spinal cord injury [30–32]. However, it has also proven somewhat unreliable in the operating room, as it can be difficult to evoke in both young and adult subjects [33].

Motor evoked potentials (MEP)

While SEPs have proven to be useful in preventing spinal cord damage in many patients undergoing high risk spinal procedures, they were not completely successful in preventing catastrophic damage to the spinal cord. This is because SEPs only assess the sensory pathways of the spinal cord. In rare instances, sensory function remains intact, while motor function is compromised, in a condition known as anterior cord syndrome [5, 34–38]. MEPs were developed in response to this shortcoming. MEPs directly assess the condition of the patient's motor system, specifically the lateral corticospinal tracts of the spinal cord, by applying a direct electrical stimulation to the patient's scalp, resulting in a stimulation of the motor cortex or the motor fibers of the internal capsule [6, 36, 37, 39–43]. Consequently, they are now considered essential for many types of spine procedures, including scoliosis and kyphosis correction surgeries, anterior corpectomies, posterior fusions for spine fractures, and spinal cord tumors [37, 40, 42, 44–54]. As it is a relatively new procedure, there is very little outcome data regarding their effectiveness in preventing spine injuries. Nevertheless, due to the fact that MEPs provide a direct assessment of the motor tracts of the spinal cord, MEPs are now routinely used during most complicated spine procedures that put the spinal cord at risk. MEPs are now considered the standard of care at many institutions [6, 41].

One other potential role of MEPs in the operating room is assessment of spinal cord motor nerve root health. MEPs have been shown to provide accurate assessment of the C5 nerve root during cervical laminectomies [47], and thus could prove useful in many types of procedures that place the C5 nerve root at risk, such as laminoplasties and anterior fusions. Neuroprotection of other specific nerve roots may prove more difficult however, due to the fact that the other muscles evaluated during MEP testing receive nerve root innervation from multiple spinal cord levels.

In the clinic, MEPs are a relatively new phenomenon and have not been heavily utilized as a clinical diagnostic tool. However, studies have shown that MEPs can be used in the clinic as an effective diagnostic tool. For example, MEPs have been shown to be an effective tool in diagnosing cervical radiculopathy [55, 56], lumbosacral spinal cord lesions [57, 58], spinal stenosis [59], and spondylotic myelopathy [56, 60, 61].

Electromyography (EMG)

EMG is a technique for evaluating muscle activity. In the operating room, spontaneous electromyography (sEMG) is used to assess the activity of the spinal cord motor nerve roots innervating a select group of muscles. These muscles are selected, depending on the procedure, to sense any perturbation on the motor nerve roots that may be placed at risk during a specific surgical procedure. Spontaneous electromyography is certainly effective at detecting impact and perturbations in motor nerve roots. However, its effectiveness at sensing nerve root injury is currently unclear.

In the clinic, EMG studies have proven to be quite useful in diagnosing and localizing spinal nerve root disorders. Fine-needle EMG studies consist of inserting a fine wire recording electrode into the belly of a muscle and recording spontaneous activity. The presence of fibrillations in the muscle may reflect spinal nerve root radiculopathies, even in the absence of imaging findings [62, 63], although such findings are, of course,

limited to motor nerve roots. Fine-needle EMG cannot detect sensory nerve root radiculopathies, which unfortunately, are commonly affected by spinal disorders such as disc herniations [10, 64–66].

As a corollary to EMG studies, nerve conduction velocity (NCV) studies are frequently done in order to rule out peripheral neuropathies affecting nerve function. Nerve conduction velocity studies specifically evaluate peripheral nerve function, distal to the spinal nerve roots. In the presence of pain, numbness, or weakness, normal NCV results point to a proximal nerve root disorder. An exception to this is for pure motor NCV studies. Abnormal results can be observed as a consequence of proximal nerve root pathology, if significant axonal loss has occurred as a result of a severe radiculopathy [67].

Finally, an important adjunct application of EMG is screw stimulation. This technique utilizes EMG recordings from muscles innervated by the relevant spinal levels being instrumented (cervical, thoracic, or lumbosacral) with electrical stimulation of a lateral mass or pedicle screw following screw placement. Utilizing increasing stimulus intensity, an electrical "threshold" is established that evokes EMG activity in the relevant muscles (if activity is evoked at all). There is well-established research evidence that a breach in the pedicle walls, which can cause nerve root irritation and iatrogenic injury, results in a substantially lower threshold (for example, <6mA) for evoked muscle activity than for a properly placed pedicle screw [68–72]. Thus a lower threshold for EMG activity indicates the need for realignment of the misplaced screw. And while there is some disagreement with regard to the stimulus threshold below which incorrect screw placement can be assumed, stimulus threshold above 15mA indicates that there is a high probability that the pedicle walls are intact [72–76].

Shortcomings

The use of electrodiagnostic techniques in spine care has increased greatly over the last decade, with more techniques being introduced in the operating room as well as the clinical setting. Physicians, surgeons, and neurophysiologists have come to rely on the results obtained from these studies for diagnosing ailments as well as planning treatment options and preventing iatrogenic injury during surgical instrumentation. In fact, it is arguable that electrodiagnostic monitoring in spine care has become so prevalent and ubiquitous that adequately evaluating the clinical relevance and impact of these techniques on outcomes has become more difficult. Surgeons and neurophysiologists rely heavily on the results obtained from electrodiagnostic studies. Consequently, implementing a controlled study, which would potentially deprive a large patient population of these diagnostic and preventative tests, has become difficult. Another impediment to such studies is the requirement for very large patient populations, in order to adequately evaluate the statistical significance of the test results. Currently, as a result, there are no controlled studies investigating the utility of electrodiagnostic testing in the clinic or in the operating room on spine outcomes, which is seen as a deficiency by some physicians and surgeons. Such studies would be extremely useful in evaluating the utility of electrodiagnostics in spine care, and would provide valuable feedback and research data that would allow the neurophysiologist to improve the tests, techniques, and results obtained. In addition, favorable results would certainly improve the position of electrodiagnostic testing in the medical field, which would most certainly lead to wider availability of the services to all patients.

In lieu of such controlled studies, neurophysiologists have relied on historical data to support the utility of electrodiagnostic testing in the operating room. Historical, retrospective studies evaluate surgical results obtained before and after the use of monitoring certain types of procedures, and can take advantage of results obtained from large patient populations generated at multiple institutions. Results from these studies have generally indicated that electrodiagnostic testing in the operating room provides significant neuroprotection [7, 8, 46, 75, 77–80], and has certainly contributed to the evolution of neuromonitoring as well as its proliferation.

The evolution of neuromonitoring has been driven by the implementation of new tests and techniques in order to evaluate spine function and condition more completely. However, despite the introduction of techniques such as MEPs and pedicle screw stimulation, one significant shortcoming of the available electrodiagnostic tests is the inadequate evaluation of the spinal cord nerve root condition at a single level intraoperatively, and provision of a reliable warning criteria for possible compromise to individual nerve root function. Currently, with the exception of the C5 nerve root [47, 79], and possibly the S1 nerve root [28, 81, 82], nerve root monitoring in the operating room evaluates 2–3 groups of nerve roots, and provides feedback related to perturbation of any of these nerve roots. At present, there is little or no predictive value to the activity observed, in terms of positive or negative outcome. In addition, sEMG monitoring probably does not adequately evaluate ischemic injury to nerve roots [47]. For procedures involving the C5 nerve root, MEPs have been demonstrated to have some predictive value regarding outcome. Such results are encouraging and suggest that further refinement of the technique may eventually allow for a better evaluation of individual motor nerve root function at other spinal cord levels.

Summary

The ultimate goal of electrophysiological monitoring is the accurate diagnosis of spinal cord pathology and the prevention of iatrogenic injury during surgery. In the past, what has driven innovation and evolution of the field has been its failings and limitations. The development of MEPs, for example, was driven by the failing of SEPs to protect motor function in some scoliosis surgeries [83–85]. Undoubtedly, any future developments and advancements in electrophysiological monitoring will follow a similar path. One of the most pressing needs in the field of electrophysiological monitoring in spine care is the refinement and improvement of segmental nerve root monitoring during surgery. Nerve root injuries are rare, but do occur in spine surgery. Current techniques are not effective at predicting and preventing these injuries. More specific MEP monitoring of the motor nerve roots, perhaps via muscle electrode placement, as well as a better understanding of the significance of EMG potentials and how they relate to injury and nerve damage are essential for improving neuroprotection of nerve root function during spine surgery. Research studies using an adequate animal model, will be necessary to achieve these goals, since as previously discussed, studies in human patients have drawbacks that would prevent a timely and comprehensive evaluation of any new techniques. Such research studies would provide additional benefits of course, since they are likely to provide further validation of the importance of electrophysiological monitoring in spine care, and thus would ultimately lead to wider availability of the services within the spine care community. While there is undeniable value in neurological monitoring during complex spinal surgery, routine usage may not improve safety and may adversely affect cost. Future efforts may be devoted to developing standards of appropriate usage in order to optimize safety and efficiency.

References

1. **Moller AR** (1988) *Evoked potentials in intraoperative monitoring.* Williams & Wilkins Company: Baltimore.
2. **Penfield W, Boldrey E** (1937) Somatic motor and sensory representation in the cerebral cortex of man as studied by electrical stimulation. *Brain;* 37:389–443.
3. **Engler GL, Spielholz NJ, Bernhard WN, et al** (1978) Somatosensory evoked potentials during Harrington instrumentation for scoliosis. *J Bone Joint Surg Am;* 60:528–532.
4. **McCallum JE, Bennett MH** (1975) Electrophysiologic monitoring of spinal cord function during intraspinal surgery. *SurgForum;* 26:469–471.
5. **Nash CL Jr, Lorig RA, Schatzinger LA, et al** (1977) Spinal cord monitoring during operative treatment of the spine. *Clin Orthop Relat Res;* 100–105.
6. **Padberg AM, Wilson-Holden TJ, Lenke LG, et al** (1998) Somatosensory- and motor-evoked potential monitoring without a wake-up test during idiopathic scoliosis surgery. An accepted standard of care. *Spine;* 23:1392–1400.
7. **Padberg AM, Russo MH, Lenke LG, et al** (1996) Validity and reliability of spinal cord monitoring in neuromuscular spinal deformity surgery. *J Spinal Disord;* 9:150–158.
8. **Nuwer MR, Dawson EG, Carlson LG, et al** (1995) Somatosensory evoked potential spinal cord monitoring reduces neurologic deficits after scoliosis surgery: results of a large multicenter survey. *Electroencephalogr Clin Neurophysiol;* 96:6–11.
9. **Egli D, Hausmann O, Schmid M, et al** (2007) Lumbar spinal stenosis: assessment of cauda equina involvement by electrophysiological recordings. *J Neurol;* 254:741–750.
10. **Beyaz EA, Akyuz G, Us O** (2009) The role of somatosensory evoked potentials in the diagnosis of lumbosacral radiculopathies. *Electromyogr Clin Neurophysiol;* 49:131–142.
11. **Haig AJ, Tong HC, Yamakawa KS, et al** (2006) Spinal stenosis, back pain, or no symptoms at all? A masked study comparing radiologic and electrodiagnostic diagnoses to the clinical impression. *Arch Phys Med Rehabil.;* 87:897–903.
12. **Liu X, Konno S, Miyamoto M, et al** (2009) Clinical usefulness of assessing lumbar somatosensory evoked potentials in lumbar spinal stenosis. Clinical article. *J Neurosurg Spine;* 11:71–78.
13. **Sitzoglou K, Fotiou F, Tsiptsios I, et al** (1997) Dermatomal SEPs—a complementary study in evaluating patients with lumbosacral disc prolapse. *Int JPsychophysiol;* 25:221–226.
14. **Tsai TM, Tsai CL, Lin TS, et al** (2005) Value of dermatomal somatosensory evoked potentials in detecting acute nerve root injury: an experimental study with special emphasis on stimulus intensity. *Spine (Phila Pa 1976);* 30:E540–E546.
15. **Righetti CA, Tosi L, Zanette G** (1996) Dermatomal somatosensory evoked potentials in the diagnosis of lumbosacral radiculopathies. *Ital J Neurol Sci;* 17:193–199.
16. **Eisen A, Hoirch M, Moll A** (1983) Evaluation of radiculopathies by segmental stimulation and somatosensory evoked potentials. *Can J Neurol Sci;* 10:178–182.
17. **Dumitru D, Dreyfuss P** (1996) Dermatomal/segmental somatosensory evoked potential evaluation of L5/S1 unilateral/unilevel radiculopathies. *Muscle Nerve;* 19:442–449.
18. **Schmid UD, Hess CW, Ludin HP** (1988) Somatosensory evoked potentials following nerve and segmental stimulation do not confirm cervical radiculopathy with sensory deficit. *J Neurol Neurosurg Psychiatry;* 51:182–187.
19. **Aminoff MJ, Goodin DS, Barbaro NM, et al** (1985) Dermatomal somatosensory evoked potentials in unilateral lumbosacral radiculopathy. *Ann Neurol;* 17:171–176.
20. **Aminoff MJ, Goodin DS, Parry GJ, et al** (1985) Electrophysiologic evaluation of lumbosacral radiculopathies: electromyography, late responses, and somatosensory evoked potentials. *Neurology;* 35:1514–1518.
21. **No authors listed** (1997) Assessment: dermatomal somatosensory evoked potentials. Report of the American Academy of Neurology's Therapeutics and Technology Assessments Subcommittee. *Neurology;* 49:1127–1130.
22. **Black S, Trankina MF** (1999) Regional anesthesia for spine surgery. *Techniques in Regional Anesthesia and Pain Management;* 3:85–93.
23. **Coscia MF, Trammell TR, Popp B, et al** (1995) Effect of anesthetic variables on dermatomal somatosensory-evoked potential monitoring in elective lumbar spinal surgery. *J Spinal Disord;* 8:451–456.
24. **Owen JH, Padberg AM, Spahr-Holland L, et al** (1991) Clinical correlation between degenerative spine disease and dermatomal somatosensory-evoked potentials in humans. *Spine (Phila Pa 1976);* 16:S201–S205.
25. **Tsai RY, Yang RS, Nuwer MR, et al** (1997) Intraoperative dermatomal evoked potential monitoring fails to predict outcome from lumbar decompression surgery. *Spine (Phila Pa 1976);* 22:1970–1975.
26. **Fisher MA** (2002) Electrophysiology of radiculopathies. *Clin Neurophysiol;* 113:317–335.
27. **Mazzocchio R** (2001) Soleus H-reflex changes during loading and unloading of the spine and their relation to the diagnosis of lumbosacral radiculopathy in mechanical back pain. *Clin Neurophysiol;* 112:1952–1954.
28. **Mazzocchio R, Scarfo GB, Cartolari R, et al** (2000) Abnormalities of the soleus H-reflex in lumbar spondylolisthesis: a possible early sign of bilateral S1 root dysfunction. *J Spinal Disord;* 13:487–495.
29. **Fisher MA** (2002) H reflexes and F waves. Fundamentals, normal and abnormal patterns. *Neurol Clin;* 20:339–360.

30. **Leis AA, Zhou HH, Mehta M, et al** (1996) Behavior of the H-reflex in humans following mechanical perturbation or injury to rostral spinal cord. *Muscle Nerve;* 19:1373–1382.

31. **Leppanen RE** (2004) From the electrodiagnostics lab: where transcranial stimulation, H-reflexes and F-responses monitor cord function intraoperatively. *Spine J;* 4:601–603.

32. **Leis AA, Kronenberg MF, Stetkarova I, et al** (1996) Spinal motoneuron excitability after acute spinal cord injury in humans. *Neurology;* 47:231–237.

33. **Devlin VJ, Anderson PA, Schwartz DM, et al** (2006) Intraoperative neurophysiologic monitoring: focus on cervical myelopathy and related issues. *Spine J;* 6:212S–224S.

34. **Van Orman CB, Darwish HZ** (1988) Harrington rod instrumentation: a cause of Brown-Sequard syndrome. *Can J Neurol Sci;* 15:44–46.

35. **Bridwell KH, Lenke LG, Baldus C, et al** (1998) Major intraoperative neurologic deficits in pediatric and adult spinal deformity patients. Incidence and etiology at one institution. *Spine (Phila Pa 1976);* 23:324–331.

36. **MacDonald DB, al Zayed Z, Khoudeir I, et al** (2003) Monitoring scoliosis surgery with combined multiple pulse transcranial electric motor and cortical somatosensory-evoked potentials from the lower and upper extremities. *Spine;* 28:194–203.

37. **Hilibrand AS, Schwartz DM, Sethuraman V, et al** (2004) Comparison of transcranial electric motor and somatosensory evoked potential monitoring during cervical spine surgery. *J Bone Joint Surg Am;* 86–A:1248–1253.

38. **Ginsburg HH, Shetter AG, Raudzens PA** (1985) Postoperative paraplegia with preserved intraoperative somatosensory evoked potentials. Case report. *J Neurosurg;* 63:296–300.

39. **Owen JH, Bridwell KH, Grubb R, et al** (1991) The clinical application of neurogenic motor evoked potentials to monitor spinal cord function during surgery. *Spine;* 16:S385–S390.

40. **MacDonald DB** (2006) Intraoperative motor evoked potential monitoring: overview and update. *J Clin Monit Comput;* 20:347–377.

41. **Pereon Y, Nguyen The Tich S, Delecrin J, et al** (1999) Somatosensory- and motor-evoked potential monitoring without a wake-up test during idiopathic scoliosis surgery: an accepted standard of care. *Spine;* 24:1169–1170.

42. **Isley MR, Balzer JR, Pearlman RC, et al** (2001) Intraoperative motor evoked potentials. *Am J END Technol;* 41:266–338.

43. **Deletis V, Isgum V, Amassian VE** (2001) Neurophysiological mechanisms underlying motor evoked potentials in anesthetized humans. Part 1. Recovery time of corticospinal tract direct waves elicited by pairs of transcranial electrical stimuli. *Clin Neurophysiol;* 112:438–444.

44. **Kothbauer KF, Novak K** (2004) Intraoperative monitoring for tethered cord surgery: an update. *Neurosurg Focus;* 16:E8.

45. **Castellon AT, Meves R, Avanzi O** (2009) Intraoperative neurophysiologic spinal cord monitoring in thoracolumbar burst fractures. *Spine (Phila Pa 1976);* 34:2662–2668.

46. **Bose B, Sestokas AK, Schwartz DM** (2004) Neurophysiological monitoring of spinal cord function during instrumented anterior cervical fusion. *Spine J.;* 4:202–207.

47. **Bose B, Sestokas AK, Schwartz DM** (2007) Neurophysiological detection of iatrogenic C-5 nerve deficit during anterior cervical spinal surgery. *J Neurosurg Spine;* 6:381–385.

48. **Gokaslan ZL, Samudrala S, Deletis V, et al** (1997) Intraoperative monitoring of spinal cord function using motor evoked potentials via transcutaneous epidural electrode during anterior cervical spinal surgery. *J Spinal Disord;* 10:299–303.

49. **Lang EW, Chesnut RM, Beutler AS, et al** (1996) The utility of motor-evoked potential monitoring during intramedullary surgery. *Anesth Analg;* 83:1337–1341.

50. **Kothbauer KF** (2007) Intraoperative neurophysiologic monitoring for intramedullary spinal-cord tumor surgery. *Neurophysiol Clin;* 37:407–414.

51. **Sala F, Palandri G, Basso E, et al** (2006) Motor evoked potential monitoring improves outcome after surgery for intramedullary spinal cord tumors: a historical control study. *Neurosurgery;* 58:1129–1143.

52. **Lee JY, Hilibrand AS, Lim MR, et al** (2006) Characterization of neurophysiologic alerts during anterior cervical spine surgery. *Spine (Phila Pa 1976);* 31:1916–1922.

53. **Neuloh G, Pechstein U, Schramm J** (2007) Motor tract monitoring during insular glioma surgery. *J Neurosurg;* 106:582–592.

54. **Legatt AD** (2002) Current practice of motor evoked potential monitoring: results of a survey. *J Clin Neurophysiol;* 19:454–460.

55. **Chistyakov AV, Soustiel JF, Hafner H, et al** (1995) Motor and somatosensory conduction in cervical myelopathy and radiculopathy. *Spine (Phila Pa 1976);* 20:2135–2140.

56. **Herdmann J, Dvorak J, Bock WJ** (1992) Motor evoked potentials in patients with spinal disorders: upper and lower motor neurone affection. *Electromyogr Clin Neurophysiol;* 32:323–330.

57. **Di LV, Pilato F, Oliviero A, et al** (2004) Role of motor evoked potentials in diagnosis of cauda equina and lumbosacral cord lesions. *Neurology;* 63:2266–2271.

58. **Machida M, Yamada T, Krain L, et al** (1991) Magnetic stimulation: examination of motor function in patients with cervical spine or cord lesion. *J Spinal Disord;* 4:123–130.

59. **Liu X, Konno S, Miyamoto M, et al** (2009) Clinical value of motor evoked potentials with transcranial magnetic stimulation in the assessment of lumbar spinal stenosis. *Int Orthop;* 33:1069–1074.

60. **Simo M, Szirmai I, Aranyi Z** (2004) Superior sensitivity of motor over somatosensory evoked potentials in the diagnosis of cervical spondylotic myelopathy. *Eur J Neurol;* 11:621–626.

61. **Travlos A, Pant B, Eisen A** (1992) Transcranial magnetic stimulation for detection of preclinical cervical spondylotic myelopathy. *Arch Phys Med Rehabil;* 73:442–446.

62. **Nasca RJ** (2009) Cervical radiculopathy: current diagnostic and treatment options. *J Surg Orthop Adv;* 18:13–18.

63. **Johnson EW, Fletcher FR** (1981) Lumbosacral radioculopathy: review of 100 consecutive cases. *Arch Phys Med Rehabil;* 62:321–323.

64. **Lee DH, Claussen GC, Oh S** (2004) Clinical nerve conduction and needle electromyography studies. *J Am Acad Orthop Surg;* 12:276–287.

65. **Nygaard OP, Mellgren SI** (1998) The function of sensory nerve fibers in lumbar radiculopathy. Use of quantitative sensory testing in the exploration of different populations of nerve fibers and dermatomes. *Spine (Phila Pa 1976);* 23:348–352.

66. **Wells MD, Meyer AP, Emley M, et al** (2002) Detection of lumbosacral nerve root compression with a novel composite nerve conduction measurement. *Spine (Phila Pa 1976);* 27:2811–2819.

67. **Pease WS, Lagattuta FP, Johnson EW** (1990) Spinal nerve stimulation in S1 radiculopathy. *Am J Phys Med Rehabil;* 69:77–80.

68. **Calancie B, Lebwohl N, Madsen P, et al** (1992) Intraoperative evoked EMG monitoring in an animal model. A new technique for evaluating pedicle screw placement. *Spine (Phila Pa 1976);* 17:1229–1235.

69. **Calancie B, Madsen P, Lebwohl N** (1994) Stimulus-evoked EMG monitoring during transpedicular lumbosacral spine instrumentation. Initial clinical results. *Spine (Phila Pa 1976);* 19:2780–2786.

70. **Shi YB, Binette M, Martin WH, et al** (2003) Electrical stimulation for intraoperative evaluation of thoracic pedicle screw placement. *Spine (Phila Pa 1976);* 28:595–601.

71. **Raynor BL, Lenke LG, Kim Y, et al** (2002) Can triggered electromyograph thresholds predict safe thoracic pedicle screw placement? *Spine (Phila Pa 1976);* 27:2030–2035.

72. **Raynor BL, Lenke LG, Bridwell KH, et al** (2007) Correlation between low triggered electromyographic thresholds and lumbar pedicle screw malposition: analysis of 4857 screws. *Spine (Phila Pa 1976);* 32:2673–2678.

73. **Bindal RK, Ghosh S** (2007) Intraoperative electromyography monitoring in minimally invasive transforaminal lumbar interbody fusion. *J Neurosurg Spine;* 6:126–132.

74. **Djurasovic M, Dimar JR, Glassman SD, et al** (2005) A prospective analysis of intraoperative electromyographic monitoring of posterior cervical screw fixation. *J Spinal Disord Tech;* 18:515–518.

75. **Alemo S, Sayadipour A** (2009) Role of intraoperative neurophysiologic monitoring in lumbosacral spine fusion and instrumentation: a retrospective study. *World Neurosurg.;* 73(1):72–76

76. **Donohue ML, Murtagh-Schaffer C, Basta J, et al** (2008) Pulse-train stimulation for detecting medial malpositioning of thoracic pedicle screws. *Spine (Phila Pa 1976);* 33:E378–E385.

77. **Dawson EG, Sherman JE, Kanim LE, et al** (1991) Spinal cord monitoring. Results of the Scoliosis Research Society and the European Spinal Deformity Society survey. *Spine;* 16:S361–S364.

78. **Lubitz SE, Keith RW, Crawford AH** (1999) Intraoperative experience with neuromotor evoked potentials. A review of 60 consecutive cases. *Spine (Phila Pa 1976);* 24:2030–2033.

79. **Fan D, Schwartz DM, Vaccaro AR, et al** (2002) Intraoperative neurophysiologic detection of iatrogenic C5 nerve root injury during laminectomy for cervical compression myelopathy. *Spine;* 27:2499–2502.

80. **Khan MH, Smith PN, Balzer JR, et al** (2006) Intraoperative somatosensory evoked potential monitoring during cervical spine corpectomy surgery: experience with 508 cases. *Spine;* 31:E105–E113.

81. **Makovec M, Benedicic M, Bosnjak R** (2006) H wave and spinal root potentials in neuromonitoring of S1 root function during evacuation of herniated disc: preliminary results. *Croat Med J;* 47:298–304.

82. **Bosnjak R, Makovec M** (2010) Neurophysiological monitoring of S1 root function during microsurgical posterior discectomy using H-reflex and spinal nerve root potentials. *Spine (Phila Pa 1976);* 35:423–429.

83. **Ben-David B, Taylor PD, Haller GS** (1987) Posterior spinal fusion complicated by posterior column injury. A case report of a false-negative wake-up test. *Spine (Phila Pa 1976);* 12:540–543.

84. **Lesser RP, Raudzens P, Luders H, et al** (1986) Postoperative neurological deficits may occur despite unchanged intraoperative somatosensory evoked potentials. *Ann Neurol;* 19:22–25.

85. **Johnston CE, Happel LT, Jr., Norris R, et al** (1986) Delayed paraplegia complicating sublaminar segmental spinal instrumentation. *J Bone Joint Surg Am;* 68:556–563.

4.2.1   Electromyography (EMG)

1   Spontaneous EMG

Description
Used to assess the activity of the spinal cord motor nerve roots innervating a select group of muscles. Depending on the procedure, these muscles are selected to detect any perturbation on the motor nerve roots that may be placed at risk during a surgical procedure.

Interpretation
Alerts the surgeon that a nerve root may be irritated at that time during surgery.

Clinical relevance
Minimizes the potential for neurological injury.

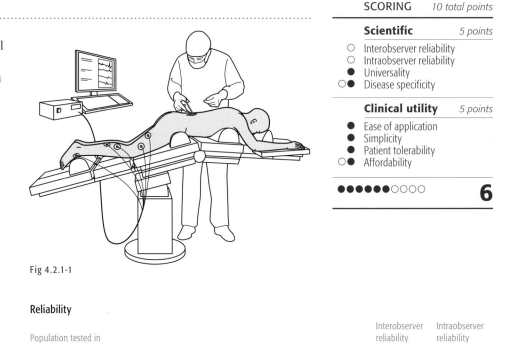

Fig 4.2.1-1

SCORING   *10 total points*

Scientific   *5 points*
○ Interobserver reliability
○ Intraobserver reliability
● Universality
○● Disease specificity

Clinical utility   *5 points*
● Ease of application
● Simplicity
● Patient tolerability
○● Affordability

●●●●●●○○○○   **6**

Reliability

Population tested in	Interobserver reliability	Intraobserver reliability
Not tested		

2   Triggered EMG

Description
The use of a stimulus electrode/Prass probe to actively stimulate soft tissue in order to identify nerve fibers within the tissue by measuring distal muscle activity.

Interpretation
Identifies and differentiates neural tissue from non-neural tissue.

Clinical relevance
Guides operative interventions based on defined neural anatomy.

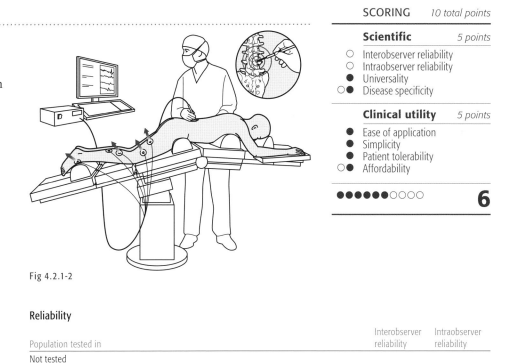

Fig 4.2.1-2

SCORING   *10 total points*

Scientific   *5 points*
○ Interobserver reliability
○ Intraobserver reliability
● Universality
○● Disease specificity

Clinical utility   *5 points*
● Ease of application
● Simplicity
● Patient tolerability
○● Affordability

●●●●●●○○○○   **6**

Reliability

Population tested in	Interobserver reliability	Intraobserver reliability
Not tested		

4.2.2   Evoked potentials

1   Somatosensory evoked potentials (SEP)

Description

Used to assess the integrity and condition of the sensory nervous system. Applied to the patient in the operating room to intraoperatively assess the condition of the spinal cord dorsal sensory columns as well as peripheral nerve function.

Interpretation

A deviation from the baseline can suggest potential spinal cord injury, or damage to peripheral nerve function (eg, brachial plexus compression or stress related to arm/shoulder position).

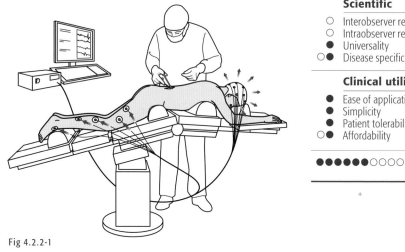

Fig 4.2.2-1

Clinical relevance

Minimizes the potential for spinal cord injury.

Reliability

Population tested in	Interobserver reliability	Intraobserver reliability
Not tested		

2   Dermatomal somatosensory evoked potentials (dSEP)

Description

Used to assess the integrity and condition of the sensory nervous system. Applied to the patient in the operating room to intraoperatively assess the condition of the spinal cord and sensory nerve roots.

Interpretation

Less commonly used and difficult to interpret intraoperatively. A deviation from the baseline can suggest potential neurological injury.

Clinical relevance

Can also be used in intraoperative and clinical settings. In a clinical setting it may provide additional information with respect to sensory radiculopathy not otherwise detected by EMG and nerve conduction velocity (NCV).

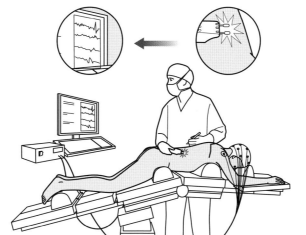

Fig 4.2.2-2

SCORING   *10 total points*

Scientific   *5 points*

○ Interobserver reliability
○ Intraobserver reliability
● Universality
○● Disease specificity

Clinical utility   *5 points*

● Ease of application
● Simplicity
● Patient tolerability
○● Affordability

●●●●●●○○○○   **6**

Reliability

Population tested in	Interobserver reliability	Intraobserver reliability
Not tested		

3   Motor evoked potentials (MEP)

Description
Used to directly assess the integrity of a patient's motor system, specifically the lateral corticospinal tracts of the spinal cord, by applying a direct electrical stimulation to the patient's scalp, resulting in the stimulation of the motor cortex or the motor fibers of the internal capsule.

Interpretation
A deviation from the baseline suggests potential spinal cord injury.

Clinical relevance
Minimizes the potential for spinal cord injury.

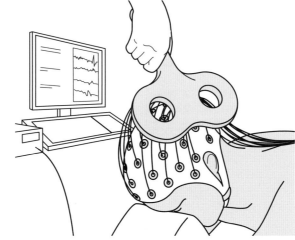

Fig 4.2.2-3

SCORING   *10 total points*

Scientific   *5 points*

○ Interobserver reliability
○ Intraobserver reliability
● Universality
○● Disease specificity

Clinical utility   *5 points*

● Ease of application
● Simplicity
● Patient tolerability
○● Affordability

●●●●●●○○○○   **6**

Reliability

Population tested in	Interobserver reliability	Intraobserver reliability
Not tested		

4   Visual evoked potentials (VEP)

Description
The measurement that results from the recordings of an electroencephalogram from the occipital area of the scalp resulting from retinal stimulation by a light flashing at quarter-second intervals, as given by a computer that averages the electroencephalogram response of 100 consecutive flashes.

Interpretation
A reduction or delay in waveform from baseline may indicate potential visual system compromise.

Generally unreliable in the operating room, due to inconsistent and variable waveforms in the presence of general anesthetic agents.

Clinical relevance
Attempts to decrease perioperative visual deficits.

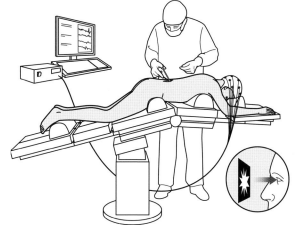

Fig 4.2.2-4

Reliability

Population tested in	Interobserver reliability	Intraobserver reliability
Not tested		

SCORING   *10 total points*

Scientific   *5 points*
- ○ Interobserver reliability
- ○ Intraobserver reliability
- ● Universality
- ●● Disease specificity

Clinical utility   *5 points*
- ○ Ease of application
- ● Simplicity
- ● Patient tolerability
- ○● Affordability

●●●●●●○○○○   **6**

4.2.3   Nerve conduction velocity (NCV)

---

1   Pedicle screw stimulation

Description
Assesses the safety of pedicle screw placement. Usually involves direct stimulation of an inserted pedicle screw to examine the threshold for evoked muscle activity.

Interpretation
In general, a threshold of greater than 10 milliamps (with pulse width of 200mA) is suggestive that the screw has been safely placed, and there is no pedicle wall breach.

Clinical relevance
Minimizes potential for neurological injury which may manifest as postoperative motor or sensory deficits.

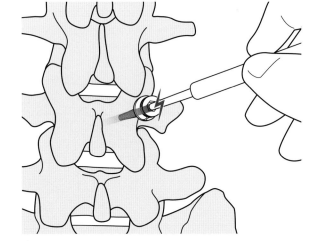

Fig 4.2.3-1

SCORING   *10 total points*

Scientific	*5 points*
○ Interobserver reliability	
○ Intraobserver reliability	
○ Universality	
○● Disease specificity	

Clinical utility	*5 points*
● Ease of application	
● Simplicity	
● Patient tolerability	
○● Affordability	

●●●●●○○○○○   **5**

Reliability

Population tested in	Interobserver reliability	Intraobserver reliability
Not tested		

2   F-waves

Description
A long latency waveform recorded in electroneuromyographical and nerve conduction tests. It appears on supramaximal stimulation of a motor nerve and is caused by antidromic transmission of a stimulus proximally to the spinal cord. The F-wave is used in studies of proximal motor nerve function in the arms and legs.

Interpretation
Absence or prolonged latencies of the F-wave, in the setting of normal nerve conduction distally, indicates a proximal peripheral nerve lesion.

Clinical relevance
Used to differentiate distal versus proximal nerve lesions.

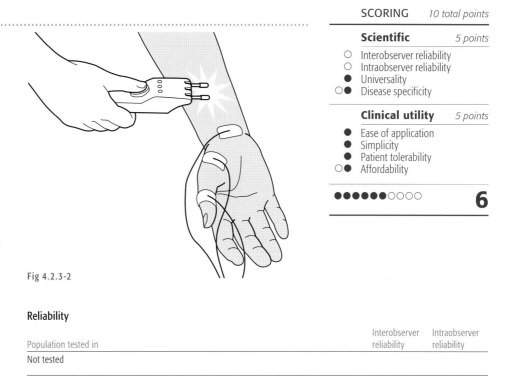

Fig 4.2.3-2

SCORING   *10 total points*

Scientific   *5 points*
- ○ Interobserver reliability
- ○ Intraobserver reliability
- ● Universality
- ○● Disease specificity

Clinical utility   *5 points*
- ● Ease of application
- ● Simplicity
- ● Patient tolerability
- ○● Affordability

●●●●●●○○○○   **6**

Reliability

Population tested in	Interobserver reliability	Intraobserver reliability
Not tested		

3   H-reflex

Description

A spinal cord reflex that involves single-level sensory nerve fibers and roots along with the complimentary motor nerve roots and fibers. Most commonly used diagnostically in the clinical setting.

Intraoperatively, the H-reflex may be modified by descending inhibitory connections; thus interruption of these connections may modify the H-reflex. Somewhat unreliable intraoperatively, and superseded by motor evoked potentials.

Stimulated bilaterally and then differentially compared.

Interpretation

Clinically, a relative weak H-reflex (as compared to contralateral side) may reflect nerve root pathology at the level of the reflex, typically at the S1 level, but may be used at the cervical (C8) level.

Intraoperatively, a change in the H-reflex may reflect spinal cord shock at a level above the injury or nerve root injury at the level of the H-reflex.

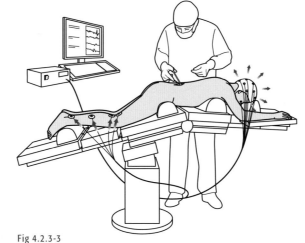

Fig 4.2.3-3

Reliability

Population tested in	Interobserver reliability	Intraobserver reliability
Not tested		

Clinical relevance

Commonly used to assess S1 nerve root pathology in a clinical setting.

Intraoperatively used to minimize the potential for spinal cord injury.

SCORING   *10 total points*

Scientific   *5 points*
○ Interobserver reliability
○ Intraobserver reliability
● Universality
○● Disease specificity

Clinical utility   *5 points*
● Ease of application
● Simplicity
● Patient tolerability
○● Affordability

●●●●●●○○○○   **6**

4   Clonus test

Description

Spasmodic alternation of muscular contraction and relaxation. Usually a sign of upper motor neuron lesion.

Interpretation

More than two beats of clonus is suggestive of an upper motor neuron lesion.

Clinical relevance

Its presence suggests spinal cord pathology or a central neurological pathology.

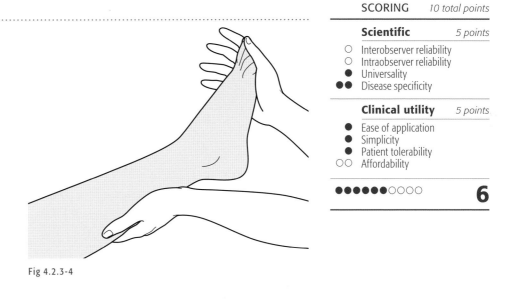

Fig 4.2.3-4

Reliability

Population tested in	Interobserver reliability	Intraobserver reliability
Not tested		

SCORING   *10 total points*

Scientific   *5 points*

○ Interobserver reliability
○ Intraobserver reliability
● Universality
●● Disease specificity

Clinical utility   *5 points*

● Ease of application
● Simplicity
● Patient tolerability
○○ Affordability

●●●●●●○○○○   **6**

5   Electroencephalogram (EEG)

Description
Technique for studying spontaneous synchronized electrical activity within the brain. Multiple scalp electrodes are placed and the synchronized activity is recorded and processed by computer software.

Interpretation
Used to assess the overall health of the brain. Certain synchronized waves are present under general anesthesia. Loss of these waves may reflect ischemic compromise to the cerebral cortex.

It can also be used to assess the level of burst suppression during certain types of brain procedures.

Clinically, used as a diagnostic and mapping tool for certain types of brain disorders such as epilepsy.

Clinical relevance
Minimizes ischemic compromise to the cerebral cortex intraoperatively.

It is a diagnostic and mapping instrument.

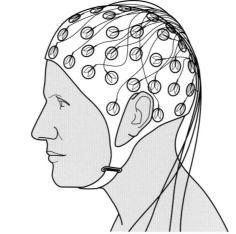

Fig 4.2.3-5

SCORING	10 total points
Scientific	5 points

○ Interobserver reliability
○ Intraobserver reliability
● Universality
○● Disease specificity

Clinical utility	5 points

● Ease of application
● Simplicity
● Patient tolerability
○● Affordability

●●●●●●○○○○   **6**

Reliability

Population tested in	Interobserver reliability	Intraobserver reliability
Not tested		

4   Laboratory measurements
4.3 Pulmonary measurements

4   Laboratory measurements

4.3   Pulmonary measurements

Introduction

Spinal disorders can influence the size, shape, and distensibility of the thoracic cage and thereby adversely impact lung function. Assessments of respiratory function include not only "lung" function, but also function of the chest wall, the diaphragm, and to a lesser extent the abdominal muscles. Scoliosis, kyphosis, and lordosis can each influence respiratory function alone, but more commonly do so together [1–3]. Loss of flexibility in the spine and costovertebral motion, such as ankylosing spondylitis, also restricts lung function [4]. In addition, spinal disorders that coexist with neuromuscular disorders, such as spasticity or weakness, adversely affect respiratory function more when concurrent than when spinal deformities exist alone [5, 6].

The influence of spinal disorders on respiratory function depends on the age of the patient. This includes the influence of spinal disorders on postnatal lung growth and function in childhood and also the progressive loss of lung function due to aging during adulthood [7]. For example, the early onset of scoliosis (beginning before 8 years of age) impacts longevity among adults after 40 years of age when lung function normally declines [8]. In growing children, spinal disorders may hinder normal postnatal lung function development such that the maximum normal values are never reached in adolescence and young adulthood. Reports concerning respiratory disorders due to spinal deformities and diseases are primarily cross-sectional descriptions of patients rather than longitudinal studies. Serial measurements of respiratory function in these patient populations may be more important than single measurements alone.

Spinal disorders produce restrictive respiratory disease much more often than obstructive lung disease [9–11]. Test results that demonstrate the presence of airway obstruction should prompt evaluation of primary lung disease and should not necessarily be attributed to spinal/thoracic cage disorders. Although central airway narrowing from torque and compression can occur as a result of scoliosis, it is an uncommon

Respiratory function

event [12, 13]. Restrictive respiratory disease is often insidious in nature and identified only when advanced. As the lungs become gradually more constrained by the spine and thorax, patients adapt such that loss of respiratory reserve goes unnoticed. Patients progressively become less active and eventually sedentary, yet breathe sufficiently well to require little medical attention. Respiratory function measurements are therefore used to assess respiratory reserve before respiratory symptoms at rest develop. Although many tests of respiratory function are performed while the patient is awake and in an outpatient setting, respiratory function during exercise and during sleep can identify abnormalities reflecting early loss of reserve [14–16].

Respiratory function can be categorized in several domains: respiratory mechanics, gas exchange, respiratory muscle function, pulmonary hemodynamics, and pulmonary host defense. Abnormalities in one domain do not always coincide with abnormalities in others. Certain tests of respiratory function are more sensitive to early respiratory changes than others. For example, restrictive lung disease with a loss of vital capacity and chest wall compliance may not lead to hypoxemia, hypercarbia, or pulmonary hypertension until spinal and chest wall deformities are severe. Changes in respiratory mechanics will occur first with spinal deformity and loss of thoracic mobility. Among the multiple measures of lung mechanics, the forced vital capacity (FVC) is the easiest to obtain in ambulatory patients repeatedly at minimal cost. The day-to-day variability of FVC values in normal children and adults is less then 10% [17]. Variability of FVC specifically among patients with scoliosis has not been reported. The FVC value reflects lung size as well as lung and chest wall distensibility and excursion.

Respiratory assessments often require voluntary efforts by patients in order to interpret tests of reserve. For example, spirometry, which includes FVC, requires an individual to inhale a maximum breath followed by a forceful rapid and complete exhalation. Patients who cannot follow instructions or who are ill, weak, or in pain, may not put forth the effort to assess respiratory function, and abnormal values will reflect inability to perform the test rather than respiratory function. Measures of respiratory muscle strength in particular are effort dependent. For this reason, respiratory assessments are usually performed in pulmonary function laboratories using equipment with specified performance criteria by technicians who are well versed in coaching patients to perform testing maneuvers [18]. Respiratory function measures in children are limited to those 5 years of age and older for this reason. Spirometry can be performed in infants 6 months to 3 years of age under sedation but only in a limited number of medical centers [19]. Some tests of respiratory function do not require exceptional effort, such as blood gas analysis, lung scans, or echocardiography, but these do not measure early respiratory changes.

There are a variety of respiratory function tests that are sensitive to early restrictive thoracic change, such as chest wall or total pulmonary compliance. These measurements, however, necessitate placement of an esophageal balloon through the nose into the esophagus. This is somewhat invasive and causes enough discomfort that it is not performed routinely in awake individuals. Chest wall compliance measurements can be performed in the operating room while the patient is sedated or anesthetized and compliance (stiffness) can be measured without active effort on the part of the patient [20, 21]. Measures of lung volume and intrathoracic pressure changes are needed to make these calculations. Importantly, serial measures of chest wall compliance in anesthetized children with scoliosis suggest that the chest wall grows stiffer with time when titanium constructs have been implanted in the chest wall [20].

Thoracoabdominal motions, in particular asynchronous movement of the chest and abdomen, have been described for patients with scoliosis [4]. Impedance belts, body netting, and reflective landmarks on the torso have been used to record relative movements of the thoraco-abdominal cylinder. In many cases, the chest wall has minimal movement and breathing depends on diaphragm and abdominal wall movement. The methods to quantify these movements and the landmarks to use across patients with abnormal thoracic configurations have not been standardized. These measurements are currently used for research purposes and not clinical decision making.

Respiratory muscle weakness predisposes patients with spine and thoracic cage disorders to low lung volumes, reduced cough effectiveness, hypoxemia during sleep, and risk for pulmonary hypertension. Muscle strength is measured easily at the bedside or in the clinic as maximum inspiratory (MIP) and maximum expiratory (MEP) pressures [22,23]. Diminished MIP values reflect either underlying muscle weakness involving the intercostal muscles and the diaphragm or, alternatively, abnormal configuration of the diaphragm, such that contraction does not produce diaphragm movement or negative intrathoracic pressure [24]. In contrast, reduced expiratory muscle strength reflects weak abdominal muscles and reduced cough effectiveness. In patients with neuromuscular weakness and scoliosis, cough peak flows below 160 liters/second place patients at risk for unsuccessful extubation [25]. Reduced MIP and MEP can also occur postoperatively due to pain and reluctance to breathe forcefully against a closed mouthpiece. Although these measurements require effort and cooperation, they are technically easy to perform and inexpensive.

Arterial oxygenation is easily measured noninvasively with the pulse oximeter, at rest, during exercise, and during sleep. The oximeter has replaced arterial blood gas sampling for partial pressure of O_2 in arterial blood (PaO_2) values. Pulse oximeters are portable and easy to use in both the medical and home setting. Capillary or arterial blood sampling remains necessary to measure partial pressure of CO_2 in arterial blood ($PaCO_2$) values, which are elevated during respiratory failure due to spinal and chest wall disease. A noninvasive way to measure partial pressure of CO_2 (PCO_2) is with a capnograph, which measures PCO_2 in exhaled breath. End-tidal PCO_2 values vary from breath to breath and can be falsely low depending on a patient's shallow breathing pattern. However, elevated levels can only be achieved with hypoventilation, and indicate hypercarbia, ie, respiratory failure. Alternatively, serum CO content, measured with electrolytes in venous blood, can be used as a surrogate for prolonged CO_2 retention, if no other reasons for metabolic alkalosis exist. The increased total CO content reflects metabolic renal compensation for persistent respiratory acidosis.

Pulmonary hypertension and cor pulmonale have been reported in adults and children with severe kyphoscoliosis [26]. However, with the advent of overnight sleep studies, known as polysomnograms (PSGs), early detection of hypoxemia, particularly during rapid eye movement (REM) sleep, has led to earlier use of home oxygen, especially at night, which prevents development of pulmonary hypertension [27]. Echocardiography is the most noninvasive and practical technique to measure right ventricular hypertrophy reflecting cor pulmonale as well as tricuspid valve and intraventricular septal motion and tricuspid jet velocity, from which pulmonary artery pressures are estimated. Pulmonary hypertension occurs prior to cor pulmonale. Echocardiograms may identify the former and not the latter when patients are screened for pulmonary vascular disease. Electrocardiograms are cheaper and more available than echocardiograms. Although they can demonstrate structural changes (eg, hypertrophy of the right ventricle) that indicate cor pulmonale, they do not detect mild to moderate pulmonary hypertension [28].

Imaging of the thorax, spine, and lung provides limited information about respiratory function. Lung volumes can be calculated from CT scans using 3-D reconstruction software [29]. Absolute lung volumes of the concave and convex lungs have been reported but may not be reproducible depending on the supine position of the patient with each measurement. In contrast, lung ventilation scans using inhaled aerosolized radio-labeled xenon, and lung perfusion scans using intravenous radio-labeled compounds demonstrate relative function of the concave and convex lungs during tidal breathing [30, 31]. This information has proven useful in conceptualizing the effect of spine rotation, chest wall deformation, and diaphragm function but has not proven its importance in clinical decision making. Dynamic MRI has demonstrated reduced diaphragm excursion in adults with scoliosis but the results depend on position and breathing pattern. The methodology has not yet been sufficiently standardized for clinical decision making [32].

Summary

Respiratory assessments are useful in detecting primary respiratory disease that may accompany spinal disease. Diagnosing and treating lung disorders is essential before addressing the spinal disease, particularly if surgical intervention is planned. Serial respiratory function measurements can also be used to assess progression of functional decline over time and to determine the short and long-term benefits of surgical interventions. Combinations of respiratory function tests may be helpful in identifying the mechanism for respiratory impairment, eg, chest wall stiffness versus respiratory muscle inefficiency versus chest wall asymmetry alone or in combinations.

Importantly, studies comparing spine and thoracic structural changes do not correlate closely with respiratory functional abnormalities [10, 30]. The three-dimensional alterations of the spine and thorax are too complex to predict function from a single structural feature, such as the Cobb angle. Consequently, assessments of structural features and various respiratory functions are used in conjunction and considered complementary measurements rather than surrogates for one another.

Tests of respiratory function yield important results that may influence clinical decision making. However, there are few reported specific thresholds of lung function that mandate intervention in everyone with a spinal disorder. Prognosis of individual patients based on respiratory functions must be couched in the context of the underlying disorder, especially as newer modes of supportive care, such as long-term noninvasive positive pressure ventilation, become available in the home setting [33, 34]. Ideally, joint collaboration between pulmonologists and spine surgeons provides additional clinical perspective for respiratory function test results and aids with clinical management of these patients.

References

1. **Dubousset J, Wicart P, Pomero V, et al** (2003) Spinal penetration index: new three-dimensional quantified reference for lordoscoliosis and other spinal deformities. *J Orthop Sci;* 8:41–49.

2. **Murray PM, Weinstein SL, Spratt KF** (1993) The natural history and long-term follow-up of Scheuermann kyphosis. *J Bone Joint Surg Am;* 75:236–248.

3. **Newton PO, Faro FD, Gollogly S, et al** (2005) Results of preoperative pulmonary function testing of adolescents with idiopathic scoliosis. A study of six hundred and thirty-one patients. *J Bone Joint Surg Am;* 87:1937–1946.

4. **Tzelepis GE, Kalliakosta G, Tzioufas AG, et al** (2009) Thoracoabdominal motion in ankylosing spongylitis: association with standardised clinical measures and response to therapy. *Ann Rheum Dis;* 68:966–971.

5. **Berven S, Bradford DS** (2002) Neuromuscular scoliosis: causes of deformity and principles for evaluation and management. *Seminars in Neurology;* 22:167–178.

6. **Sherman MS, Kaplan JM, Effgen S, et al** (1997) Pulmonary dysfunction and reduced exercise capacity in patients with myelomeningocele. *J Pediatr;* 131:413–418.

7. **Knudson RJ, Clark DF, Kennedy TC, et al** (1977) Effect of aging alone on mechanical properties of the normal adult human lung. *J Appl Physiol;* 43:1054–1062.

8. **Pehrsson K, Danielsson A, Nachemson A** (2001) Pulmonary function in adolescent idiopathic scoliosis: a 25 year follow up after surgery or start of brace treatment. *Thorax;* 56:388–393.

9. **Day GA, Upadhyay SS, Ho EKW, et al** (1994) Pulmonary functions in congenital scoliosis. *Spine;* 19:1027–1031.

10. **Mayer OH, Redding G** (2009) Early changes in pulmonary function after vertical expandable prosthetic titanium rib insertion in children with thoracic insufficiency syndrome. *J Pediatr Orthop;* 29:35–38.

11. **Owange-Iraka JW, Harrison A, Warner JO** (1984) Lung function in congenital and idiopathic scoliosis. *Eur J Pediatr;* 142:198–200.

12. **Al-Kattan K, Simonds A, Chung KF, et al** (1997) Kyphoscoliosis and bronchial torsion. *Chest;* 111:1134–1137.

13. **Boyer J, Amin N, Taddonio R, et al** (1996) Evidence of airway obstruction in children with idiopathic scoliosis. *Chest;* 109:1532–1535.

14. **Barrios C, Perez–Encinas D, Maruenda JI, et al** (2005) Significant ventilatory functional restriction in adolescents with mild or moderate scoliosis during maximal exercise tolerance test. *Spine;* 30:1610–1615.

15. **Smyth RJ, Chapman KR, Wright TA, et al** (1986) Ventilatory patterns during hypoxia, hypercapnia, and exercise in adolescents with mild scoliosis. *Pediatrics;* 77:692–697.

16. **Yuan N, Skaggs DL, Davidson Ward SL, et al** (2004) Preoperative polysomnograms and infant pulmonary function tests do not predict prolonged postoperative mechanical ventilation in children following scoliosis repair. *Pediatr Pulmonol;* 38:256–260.

17. **Nickerson BG, Lemen RJ, Gerdes CB, et al** (1980) Within-subject variability and per cent change for significance of spirometry in normal subjects and in patients with cystic fibrosis. *Am Rev Respir Dis;* 122:859–866.

18. **Miller MR, Hankinson J, Brusasco V, et al** (2005) Standardisation of spirometry. *Eur Respir J;* 26:319–338.

19. **Castile R, Filbrun D, Flucke R, et al** (2000) Adult-type pulmonary function tests in infants without respiratory disease. *Pediatr Pulmonol;* 30:215–227.

20. **Motoyama EK, Yang CI, Deeney VF** (2009) Thoracic malformation with early-onset scoliosis: Effect of serial VEPTR expansion thoracoplasty on lung growth and function in children. *Paediatr Respir Rev;* 10:12–17.

21. **Motoyama EK, Deeney VF, Fine GF, et al** (2006) Effects of lung function of multiple expansion thoracoplasty in children with Thoracic Insufficiency Syndrome: *A longitudinal study. Spine;* 31:284–290.

22. **Lisboa C, Moreno R, Fava M, et al** (1985) Inspiratory muscle function in patients with severe kyphoscoliosis. *Am Rev Respir Dis;* 132:48–52.

23. **Szeinberg A, Canny GJ, Rashed N, et al** (1988) Forced vital capacity and maximal respiratory pressures in patients with mild and moderate scoliosis. *Pediatr Pulmonol;* 4:8–12.

24. **Giordano A, Fuso L, Galli M, et al** (1997) Evaluation of pulmonary ventilation and diaphragmatic movement in idiopathic scoliosis using radioaerosol ventilation scintigraphy. *Nuclear Medicine Communications;* 18:105–111.

25. **King M, Brock G, Lundell C** (1985) Clearance of mucus by simulated cough. *J Appl Physiol;* 58:1776–1782.

26. **Primiano FP, Nussbaum E, Hirschfeld SS, et al** (1983) Early echocardiographic and pulmonary function findings in idiopathic scoliosis. *J Pediatr Orthop;* 3:475–481.

27. **Striegl A, Chen M, Kifle Y, et al** (2010) Sleep-related breathing disorders in children with thoracic insufficiency syndrome. *Pediatr Pulmonol;* 45(5):469–474.

28. **Schannwell CM, Steiner S, Strauer BE** (2007) Diagnostics in pulmonary hypertension. *J Physiol Pharmacol;* Suppl 5:591–602.

29. **Gollogly S, Smith JT, White SK, et al** (2004) The volume of lung parenchyma as a function of age: a review of 1050 normal CT scans of the chest with three-dimensional volumetric reconstruction of the pulmonary system. *Spine;* 29:2061–2066.

30. **Redding G, Song K, Inscore S, et al** (2007) Lung function asymmetry in children with congenital and infantile scoliosis. *Spine;* 8:639–644.

31. **Padua R, Ceccarelli E, Pitta L, et al** (2002) Radioaerosol lung scintigraphy in idiopathic scoliosis. *Tanguy A, Peuchot B (eds), Research into Spinal Deformities* 3rd ed. Amsterdam: IOS Press, 279–283.

32. **Kotani T, Minami S, Takahashi K, et al**
    (2004) An analysis of chest wall and
    diaphragm motions in patients with idiopathic
    scoliosis using dynamic breathing MRI. *Spine;*
    29:298–302.
33. **Ferris G, Servera-Pieras E, Vergara P, et al**
    (2000) Kyphoscoliosis ventilatory insufficiency:
    noninvasive management outcomes. *Am J
    Phys Med Rehabil;* 79:24–29.
34. **Fuschillo S, De Felice A, Gaudiosi C, et al**
    (2003) Nocturnal mechanical ventilation
    improves exercise capacity in kyphoscoliotic
    patients with respiratory impairment. *Monaldi
    Arch Chest Dis;* 59:281–286.

4.3.1 Lung mechanics

---

1   Lung and chest wall compliance

Description
Ability of the lungs to stretch during a change in volume relative to an applied change in pressure.

Interpretation
Change in esophageal and mouth pressure differences, with changes in known volumes into or out of the chest. Done primarily in the operating room or under sedation.

Clinical relevance
Not a routine clinical test. Used for research purposes.

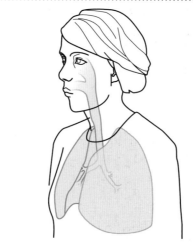

Fig 4.3.1-1

SCORING   *10 total points*

Scientific   *5 points*
- ○ Interobserver reliability
- ○ Intraobserver reliability
- ● Universality
- ○● Disease specificity

Clinical utility   *5 points*
- ● Ease of application
- ○ Simplicity
- ○ Patient tolerability
- ○● Affordability

●●●●○○○○○○   **4**

Reliability

Population tested in	Interobserver reliability	Intraobserver reliability
Not tested		

2   Spirometry

Description
Measurement of the amount (volume) and/or speed (flow) of air that can be inhaled and exhaled.

The spirometry test is performed using a device called a spirometer, which comes in several different varieties.

Interpretation
Spirometers display the following graphs, called spirograms:
- A volume-time curve, showing volume (liters) along the Y-axis and time (seconds) along the X-axis
- A flow-volume loop that graphically depicts the rate of airflow on the Y-axis and the total volume inspired or expired on the X-axis

Clinical relevance
Distinguishes restrictive from obstructive abnormalities. Monitors changes in forced vital capacity (FVC) serially for changes in restrictive lung/chest wall disease. Uses forced expiratory volume in 1 second (FEV1) divided by FVC to assess obstructive airway disease (FEVI/FVC).

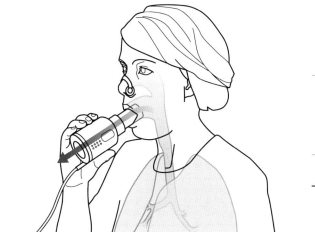

Fig 4.3.1-2

Reliability

Population tested in	Interobserver reliability	Intraobserver reliability
Not tested		

SCORING   *10 total points*

Scientific   *5 points*
- ○ Interobserver reliability
- ○ Intraobserver reliability
- ● Universality
- ○● Disease specificity

Clinical utility   *5 points*
- ● Ease of application
- ● Simplicity
- ● Patient tolerability
- ●● Affordability

●●●●●●●○○○   **7**

3   Gas dilution

Description
Method of determining lung volume that cannot be determined by spirometry. These include:
- Functional residual capacity (FRC)
- Residual volume (RV)
- Total lung capacity (TLC)

Interpretation
FRC is the sum of the expiratory reserve volume (ERV) and residual volume (RV) and measures approximately 2.4 L/1.9 L in an average sized male/female.

RV is the volume of air remaining in the lungs after maximal expiratory effort and measures approximately 1.2 L/0.93 L in an average sized male/female.

TLC is the volume of air contained in the lung at the end of maximal inspiration and measures approximately 6.0 L/4.7 L in an average sized male/female.

Clinical relevance
Determines presence and degree of volume loss due to restrictive lung disease (reduced TLC) and/or increased air trapping due to obstructive airway disease (increased RV).

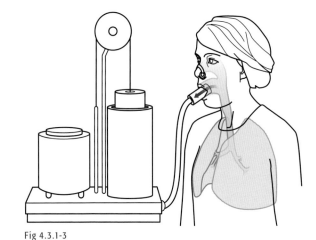

Fig 4.3.1-3

Scientific   *5 points*
- ○ Interobserver reliability
- ○ Intraobserver reliability
- ● Universality
- ●● Disease specificity

Clinical utility   *5 points*
- ● Ease of application
- ● Simplicity
- ○ Patient tolerability
- ○● Affordability

●●●●●●○○○○   **6**

Reliability

Population tested in	Interobserver reliability	Intraobserver reliability
Not tested		

4 Thoracoabdominal motion (chest wall-abdominal asynchrony)

Description

Impedance monitors placed on or around the chest and abdomen determine the relative motion of the chest wall and abdomen, and the synchrony of their movements.

Interpretation

Out-of-phase movements (paradoxical breathing) reflect respiratory muscle fatigue or weakness. Relative movements of the chest wall and abdomen are research measures.

Clinical relevance

Limited application clinically.

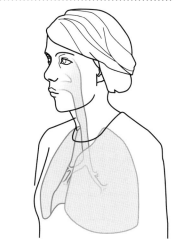

Fig 4.3.1-4

SCORING	10 total points
Scientific	5 points

○ Interobserver reliability
○ Intraobserver reliability
○ Universality
○● Disease specificity

Clinical utility	5 points

● Ease of application
● Simplicity
● Patient tolerability
○● Affordability

●●●●●○○○○○ **5**

Reliability

Population tested in	Interobserver reliability	Intraobserver reliability
Not tested		

4.3.2   Gas exchange

1   PCO$_2$ levels

Description
Sampled from venous, capillary, and arterial blood and/or exhaled breath.

Scientific   *5 points*
- ○ Interobserver reliability
- ○ Intraobserver reliability
- ● Universality
- ●● Disease specificity

Interpretation
Elevated levels represent hypoventilation and usually respiratory failure (acute or chronic).

Clinical utility   *5 points*
- ● Ease of application
- ● Simplicity
- ● Patient tolerability
- ○● Affordability

Clinical relevance
Detection of acute or chronic respiratory failure.

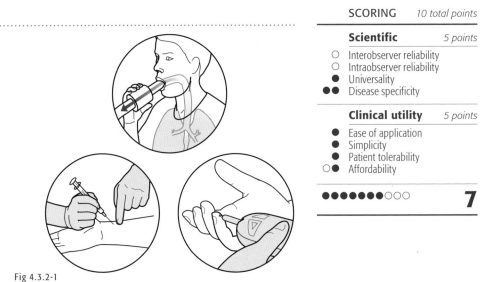

●●●●●●●○○○   **7**

Fig 4.3.2-1

Reliability

Population tested in	Interobserver reliability	Intraobserver reliability
Not tested		

2   Serum HCO₃ levels

Description
Sampled from venous blood.

Interpretation
Reflection of acid-base status including both metabolic and respiratory components. In the absence of metabolic disorders, elevated HCO_3 (also known as total CO_2 content) represents metabolic (renal) compensation for subacute or chronic CO_2 retention due to hypoventilation.

Clinical relevance
Detection of metabolic and/or respiratory disorders.

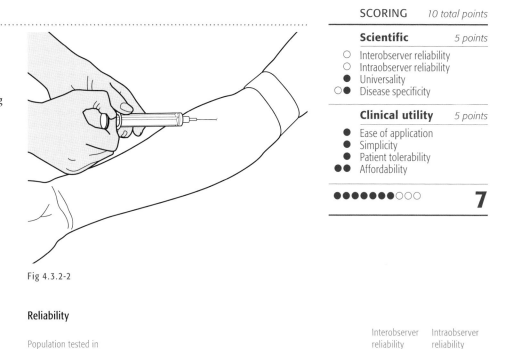

Fig 4.3.2-2

SCORING	10 total points
Scientific	5 points

○ Interobserver reliability
○ Intraobserver reliability
● Universality
○● Disease specificity

Clinical utility	5 points

● Ease of application
● Simplicity
● Patient tolerability
●● Affordability

●●●●●●●○○○   **7**

Reliability

Population tested in	Interobserver reliability	Intraobserver reliability
Not tested		

3   PaO₂ levels

Description
Sampled from arterial blood.

Interpretation
Reflects blood oxygenation and relative efficiency of the lung to oxygenate the blood. Altered by treatment with supplemental oxygen. Has been supplanted by pulse oximetry outside the intensive care unit or operating room setting.

Clinical relevance
Determines level of oxygenation of the blood by the lungs.

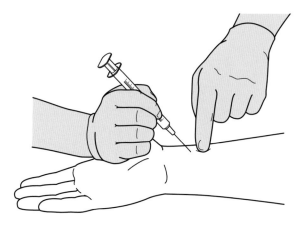

Fig 4.3.2-3

SCORING   10 total points

Scientific   5 points
○ Interobserver reliability
○ Intraobserver reliability
● Universality
○● Disease specificity

Clinical utility   5 points
● Ease of application
● Simplicity
○ Patient tolerability
○○ Affordability

●●●●○○○○○○   **4**

Reliability

Population tested in	Interobserver reliability	Intraobserver reliability
Not tested		

4   SaO₂ levels

Description
Noninvasive measure of the saturation of hemoglobin by oxygen in arterial blood. Depends on relative transmission of light of different wavelengths through an appendage such as a finger, toe, ear lobe, or nose.

Interpretation
Ongoing or intermittent assessment of blood oxygenation by the lung (in the absence of congenital heart disease).

Clinical relevance
Bedside assessment of oxygenation of blood used in the inpatient, outpatient, and home settings.

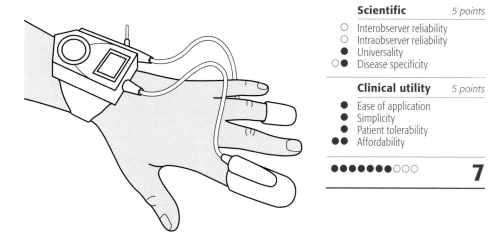

Fig 4.3.2-4

SCORING	10 total points
Scientific	5 points

○ Interobserver reliability
○ Intraobserver reliability
● Universality
○● Disease specificity

Clinical utility	5 points

● Ease of application
● Simplicity
● Patient tolerability
●● Affordability

●●●●●●●○○○   **7**

Reliability

Population tested in	Interobserver reliability	Intraobserver reliability
Not tested		

4.3.3   Regional lung function

1   Lung ventilation scans

Description
Medical imaging that uses scintigraphy and medical isotopes to evaluate the circulation of air within the patient's lungs.

Measures the ability of air to reach all parts of the lungs.

Interpretation
Determines which areas of the lungs are capable of ventilation. Can also be used to assess heterogeneity and distribution of lung function throughout the lungs.

Clinical relevance
Determines the relative contribution of the right and left lung to total ventilation. Identifies focal defects in ventilation due to regional lung disease.

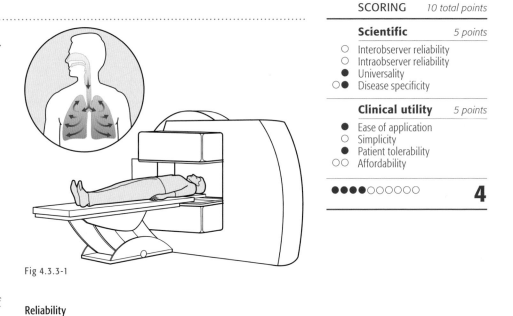

Fig 4.3.3-1

SCORING	10 total points
Scientific	5 points

- ○ Interobserver reliability
- ○ Intraobserver reliability
- ● Universality
- ○● Disease specificity

Clinical utility	5 points

- ● Ease of application
- ○ Simplicity
- ● Patient tolerability
- ○○ Affordability

●●●●○○○○○○   **4**

Reliability

Population tested in	Interobserver reliability	Intraobserver reliability
Not tested		

2 Perfusion scans

Description
Medical imaging that uses scintigraphy and medical isotopes to evaluate the circulation of blood within the patient's lungs.

Evaluates how well blood circulates within the lungs.

Interpretation
Determine the relative lung perfusion of different lung regions, eg, left versus right lung. Identifies focal reductions in lung perfusion due to lung or pulmonary vascular disease, eg, thrombosis or embolus.

Clinical relevance
Determines the relative contribution of the right and left lung to total lung perfusion. Identifies focal deficits in lung perfusion in different lung regions.

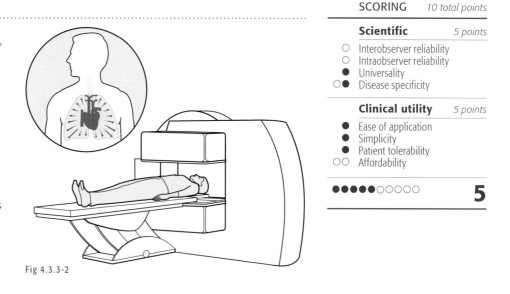

Fig 4.3.3-2

SCORING	10 total points
Scientific	5 points
○ Interobserver reliability	
○ Intraobserver reliability	
● Universality	
○● Disease specificity	
Clinical utility	5 points
● Ease of application	
● Simplicity	
● Patient tolerability	
○○ Affordability	

●●●●●○○○○○ **5**

Reliability

Population tested in	Interobserver reliability	Intraobserver reliability
Not tested		

4.3.4   Respiratory muscle function

1   Maximum inspiratory pressure (MIP)

Description
The maximum pressure at the mouth generated by all inspiratory respiratory muscles at functional residual capacity and residual lung volume.

Interpretation
Normal value varies with age and sex. Pressures less than $-60\,cm\,H_2O$ suggest inspiratory muscle weakness or fatigue.

Clinical relevance
Determines inspiratory muscle force capabilities and conditions of muscle weakness. The measure is effort dependent.

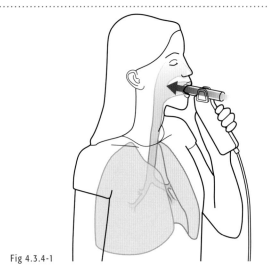

Fig 4.3.4-1

SCORING   *10 total points*

Scientific   *5 points*
○ Interobserver reliability
○ Intraobserver reliability
● Universality
●● Disease specificity

Clinical utility   *5 points*
● Ease of application
● Simplicity
● Patient tolerability
○● Affordability

●●●●●●●○○○   **7**

Reliability

Population tested in	Interobserver reliability	Intraobserver reliability
Not tested		

2   Maximum expiratory pressure (MEP)

Description
The maximum pressure at the mouth generated by all respiratory muscles. Measured as total lung capacity and less often functional residual capacity.

Interpretation
Normal value varies with age and sex. Pressures of less than +60 cm H_2O suggest expiratory, eg, abdominal muscle or generalized muscle weakness.

Clinical relevance
Identifies abdominal muscle weakness and/or generalized muscle weakness. The measure is effort dependent.

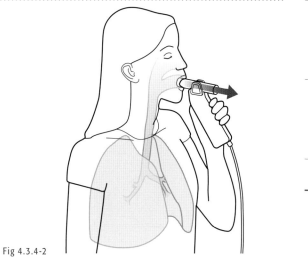

Fig 4.3.4-2

SCORING   *10 total points*

Scientific   *5 points*
○ Interobserver reliability
○ Intraobserver reliability
● Universality
○● Disease specificity

Clinical utility   *5 points*
● Ease of application
● Simplicity
● Patient tolerability
○● Affordability

●●●●●●○○○○   **6**

Reliability

Population tested in	Interobserver reliability	Intraobserver reliability
Not tested		

4.3.5   Pulmonary hemodynamics

1   Echocardiograms (ECHO)

Description
Sonographic imaging providing
noninvasive assessment of cardiac
structures, motions, dimensions, and
estimates of cardiac performance (eg,
ejection fractions). Can also assess
thickening of the right ventricle
reflecting cor pulmonale and can
estimate pulmonary artery pressures
by measuring triscupid jet velocities.

Interpretation
Assesses cardiac anatomy, function,
and adaptive changes, eg, atrial or
ventricular hypertrophy or
enlargement and pulmonary artery
pressures.

Clinical relevance
Rule out congenital heart disease,
diagnose cor pulmonale and
pulmonary hypertension. Can also
assess cardiac function.

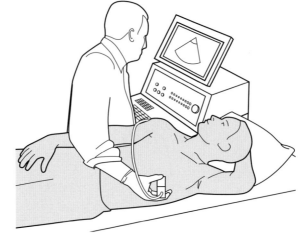

Fig 4.3.5-1

SCORING	10 total points
Scientific	5 points

○ Interobserver reliability
○ Intraobserver reliability
● Universality
●● Disease specificity

Clinical utility	5 points

● Ease of application
● Simplicity
● Patient tolerability
○● Affordability

●●●●●●●○○○   **7**

Reliability

Population tested in	Interobserver reliability	Intraobserver reliability
Not tested		

4.3.6 Pulmonary host defenses

1 Peak cough flows (PCF)

Description
Measured by using a peak flow meter. The PCF is the velocity of air being expelled from the lungs during a cough maneuver.

Interpretation
This airflow measurement is measured at the mouth and expressed in L/min. It is the maximum transient flow produced by an expulsive maneuver such as a cough.

Clinical relevance
Used to assess respiratory muscle force and airway caliber that dictate flow during a cough.

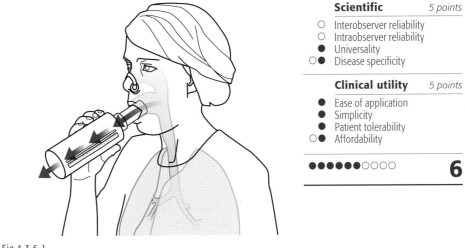

Fig 4.3.6-1

SCORING	10 total points
Scientific	5 points
○ Interobserver reliability	
○ Intraobserver reliability	
● Universality	
○● Disease specificity	
Clinical utility	5 points
● Ease of application	
● Simplicity	
● Patient tolerability	
○● Affordability	

●●●●●●○○○○ **6**

Reliability

Population tested in	Interobserver reliability	Intraobserver reliability
Not tested		

4.3.7   Response to exercise

---

1   Treadmill ergometry

....

Description

A treadmill with an ergometer to measure the cardiopulmonary performance of a person in response to external work (treadmill speed and ramp angle).

Interpretation

Measures cardiopulmonary response to external work (exercise) and degree of conditioning.

Clinical relevance

Determines cardiac and pulmonary performance in response to different levels of external work while walking or running on a treadmill.

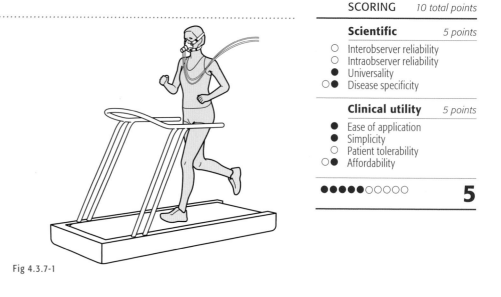

Fig 4.3.7-1

SCORING	10 total points

Scientific	5 points
○ Interobserver reliability	
○ Intraobserver reliability	
● Universality	
○● Disease specificity	

Clinical utility	5 points
● Ease of application	
● Simplicity	
○ Patient tolerability	
○● Affordability	

●●●●●○○○○○   **5**

Reliability

Population tested in	Interobserver reliability	Intraobserver reliability
Not tested		

2   Bicycle ergometry

Description
A stationary bicycle with an ergometer to measure the cardiopulmonary response to external work (produced by pedaling rate and resistance to pedaling).

Interpretation
Measures cardiopulmonary responses to external work and any limitations in exercise due to heart or pulmonary disorders or to deconditioning.

Clinical relevance
Identifies limitations in exercise due to cardiac disorders, pulmonary disorders, or abnormalities of exercising muscles.

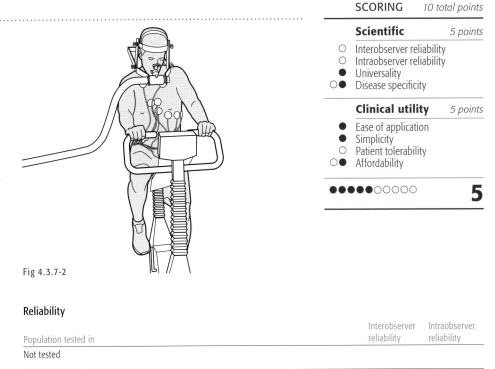

Fig 4.3.7-2

Reliability

Population tested in	Interobserver reliability	Intraobserver reliability
Not tested		

SCORING   *10 total points*

Scientific   *5 points*
○ Interobserver reliability
○ Intraobserver reliability
● Universality
○● Disease specificity

Clinical utility   *5 points*
● Ease of application
● Simplicity
○ Patient tolerability
○● Affordability

●●●●●○○○○○   **5**

4.3.8   Respiratory function during sleep

1   Polysomnography/sleep fragmentation related to hypoxemia

Description
Coordinated measurements of sleep states (electroencephalographic and muscle movement measurements) and cardiopulmonary functions during sleep. These include measures of apnea, hypoventilation, hypoxemia, and CO_2 retention.

Interpretation
Interpretation includes adequacy and quality of sleep (ie, sleep fragmentation), evidence of obstructive or central apnea, level of oxygenation and ventilation during sleep, and muscle activity which may reflect metabolic disorders, eg, restless legs syndrome. Respiratory outcomes are measured with the Apnea-Hypopnea index (AHI) in events/hour.

Clinical relevance
Determines the adequacy and nature of sleep as well as relevant etiologies behind compromised sleep.

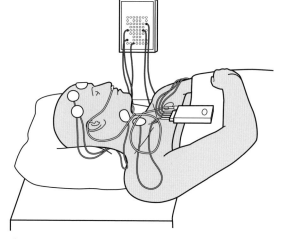

Fig 4.3.8-1

SCORING   10 total points

Scientific	5 points
○	Interobserver reliability
○	Intraobserver reliability
●	Universality
●●	Disease specificity

Clinical utility	5 points
●	Ease of application
●	Simplicity
●	Patient tolerability
○●	Affordability

●●●●●●●○○○   **7**

Reliability

Population tested in	Interobserver reliability	Intraobserver reliability
Not tested		

5   Radiographic measurements
5.1   Fractures/dislocations

5   Radiographic measurements

5.1   Fractures/dislocations

Introduction

Most spinal trauma can be treated nonoperatively, however determining which injuries are stable and which ones are unstable can be difficult. Various imaging modalities are used including plain x-rays with dynamic views, helical or axial CT scans with sagittal and coronal reformations, and MRI with various sequences. Each has its role and utility in clarifying the severity of spinal trauma and in helping determine appropriate management. Unfortunately, the interpretation of these modalities is still not uniformly agreed upon. Therefore, clinicians continue to disagree on what defines a stable injury that can be treated nonoperatively, versus what defines an unstable injury that can be treated surgically.

The evolution of imaging has allowed for a better understanding of injuries and a lower "miss rate". Plain x-rays, though helpful, are not sufficient to identify all injuries, particularly those at the craniocervical or the cervicothoracic junctions. Helical CT scans have largely replaced plain x-rays and tomography in identifying and classifying injuries, particularly in those deemed to be at high risk [1–3]. Computed tomography is more sensitive than plain x-rays, however, the responsibility of interpreting the images and identifying unstable injuries still falls on the treating clinician. Various measurements have been described in the literature to identify and classify injuries and to determine severity.

The spine, with respect to trauma, is usually separated into four primary regions:

- Upper cervical, including the craniocervical junction
- Subaxial
- Thoracic and lumbar
- Lumbosacral junction and sacral

Each region has unique injuries specific to its anatomy. As a result, different radiographic assessment tools have been developed for the individual areas.

Craniocervical junction

The craniocervical junction is composed of the occiput to the inferior aspect of C2 and has unique injuries specific to the skull base, atlas, and axis. Injuries to this junction include but are not limited to craniocervical dislocations (CCD), C1 ring fractures, transverse atlantal ligament (TAL) injuries, rotatory subluxations, dens fractures, hangman fractures, and C2 body fractures. Many of these can be difficult to diagnose on plain x-rays, therefore CT scanning is the diagnostic mode of choice as an initial screening tool for patients thought to be at risk. The common yet unique and specific radiological measurements to this region include:

• Power's ratio
• Harris lines
• C1/2 lateral mass overhang (Rule of Spence)
• Atlantodens interval (ADI)
• Atlantoaxial rotation
• Disc angulation and translation
• Prevertebral soft-tissue swelling
• C1–3 laminar line

CCDs are uncommon injuries and historically have had delayed diagnosis [4]. Of the many screening measurements, the Power's ratio, which relates the distance between basion and posterior arch of the atlas (BC) and the distance between anterior arch of the atlas and opisthion (AO), has been considered the standard for many years [5]. This Power's ratio (BC/AO) should be less than 1 in normal cases. This tool, however, is limited by being valid only for anterior atlantooccipital dislocation (AOD) cases. In the case of a longitudinal distraction or when the head is displaced posteriorly, this screening tool inherently bears no relevance. Other measurements such as Lee's lines [6], no longer have a role in the radiographic diagnosis of CCD. The accuracy of both these measurements is limited due to the difficulty of accurately identifying the basion and opisthion on the lateral cervical x-ray.

More recently, Harris refined the dens-basion interval (DBI) and added the axis-basion interval (ABI) [7, 8]. Both, the ABI and the DBI should remain less than 12 mm in 95% of adults ("rule of twelves"). He demonstrated a higher degree of specificity and sensitivity in detecting AOD with this method compared to Power's ratio. These Harris lines also have limitations and may miss serious CCD injuries in which there is disruption with a "rebound phenomenon". In the diagnosis of CCDs, subtle findings such as a type I dens fractures, anterior C1 transverse ring fractures, type III occipital condyle fractures, occiput-C1 joint incongruity, and precervical soft-tissue swelling may be indicative of a more serious underlying CCD. MRI and occasionally traction tests under fluoroscopy may ultimately be indicated. Other craniocervical measurements used for degenerative or rheumatoid conditions such as Chamberlain's line or McRae's line have no substantial role in trauma.

The Rule of Spence and ADI are largely measures that have come about in an attempt to assess for TAL competence. According to Spence, loss of structural properties of the TAL can be expected when the combined overhang of the lateral masses of the atlas extends more than 6.9 mm beyond the lateral masses of the axis [9]. Their findings have more recently been challenged by Dickman et al [10], who claimed that the 7 mm criteria would have detected only 39% of atlas fractures with disrupted transverse atlantal ligaments if x-rays alone were used. Dickman concluded that the 7 mm criterion was insensitive and inaccurate as a screening tool.

The ADI is another measurement that may suggest C1/2 instability secondary to a TAL injury. This should be less than 3 mm in an adult and less than 4.5 mm in a child [11]. Although the ADI is useful as a guide, flexion-extension x-rays are required to fully assess this instability and many patients cannot cooperate in the acute setting due to pain, confounding injuries, or mental status.

Rotatory atlantoaxial subluxation is more commonly seen in children and is usually not associated with a traumatic event. This injury is optimally assessed by evaluating the C1 to C2 joint relationship on axial CT images. Rotatory subluxation is usually misdiagnosed if the patient's head position is not taken into account. Frequently, left and right rotation CT scans are required to confirm rotatory atlantoaxial subluxation versus normal rotational position of the C1/2 joints.

Other helpful measures of the craniocervical junction include disc angulation, disc translation, prevertebral soft-tissue swelling, and C1–3 laminar line. There are no absolute numbers, and interpretation of these values can be variable. Many patients with traumatic injuries may have underlying spondylosis hence making these rules slightly arbitrary. They are better interpreted on an individual case basis. White and Panjabi are renowned for their work in determining spinal stability. They have proposed that greater than 3.5 mm of horizontal displacement or more than 11° of rotational difference of one vertebra relative to an adjacent vertebra measured on a lateral roentgenogram (resting or dynamic) constitutes an unstable segment [12].

Prevertebral soft-tissue swelling is also a helpful hint of an occult injury at the craniocervical junction. However, absolute measurements of the prevertebral soft tissues are not accurate and vary with head position, body habitus, phase of inspiration, and the presence of tracheal and esophageal tubes. These numbers vary based on levels of sensitivity and specificity, but a rough rule of thumb often used is 6 mm at C2 and 2 cm at C6. The initial measurements as initially advocated by Matar and Doyle suggest a measurement of ≥ 7 mm at C2/3 and > 21 mm at C6/7 were considered abnormal [13].

Measurement of the C1–3 spinolaminar line should find the C2 laminar line within 2 mm of the AP plane of this line. Offsets of more than 2 mm indicate malalignment of the posterior elements as found in hangman's fractures.

In addition to the discussed measurements, one must also assess displacement, angulation, and height loss in determining stability. There are no specific rules for displacement for most fractures of the craniocervical junction except for displacement and angulation as those pertaining to dens fractures. For dens fractures through the waist of the dens (type II), most advocate that > 5 mm of displacement or > 11° of angulation represent an unstable fracture.

Subaxial cervical spine

Common injuries of the subaxial spine include axial load compression or burst injuries, flexion-distraction type injuries with facet fractures or dislocations, extension injuries, and lamina, spinous process, or transverse process fractures.

Whereas the craniocervical junction has numerous specific measurements that may be useful, the subaxial spine does not. The main lines used in evaluating the subaxial cervical spine are that of alignment (along the anterior and posterior longitudinal ligaments, facets, lamina and spinous processes), disc height, and angulation to identify injuries. The location of the fracture, the mechanism of injury, and the amount of displacement help determine instability. As mentioned previously, White and Panjabi have suggested that more than 3.5 mm of horizontal displacement or more than 11° of rotation of one vertebra relative to an adjacent vertebra constitutes an unstable segment [12]. This is a reasonable guideline but must be taken in the context of the individual patient's baseline cervical spondylosis.

The goal is to differentiate stable from unstable when there are very few reliable, specific radiographic measurements. One can measure displacement, angulation, height loss, and facet gapping, but then must decide overall whether the injury is stable with few reliable specific rules.

Current guidelines suggest that cervical spine immobilization be continued for awake patients with neck tenderness and normal cervical spine x-rays and/or CT scans until either adequate flexion/extension x-rays can be obtained or an MRI can be obtained [14]. However, it may be difficult to obtain acceptable flexion/extension x-rays in up to 33% of patients with neck pain and stiffness [15, 16]. These dynamic studies sometimes need to be delayed up to two weeks after the initial trauma until acceptable motion and excursion can be obtained. In patients undergoing flexion/extension x-rays, the aim is to look for instability with translation greater than 3.5 mm or a change in angulation of more than 11° between adjacent vertebral levels [12].

More recent studies have advocated that CT scans alone are adequate and should not miss even subtle ligamentous injuries in the obtunded patient, and therefore, flexion/extension x-rays may no longer be necessary [17–19]. Other studies suggest that CT alone is not sufficient in trauma patients and an MRI or flexion/extension x-rays are necessary to assess for subtle injuries [20]. One recent study proposed that flexion/extension x-rays are still necessary, even if CT and MRI scans are interpreted as being negative [21]. Thus, there is an ongoing debate as to the utility and indications of dynamic x-rays in the trauma population. Most would advocate that this imaging modality still plays an important role in assessing stability.

Thoracolumbar and lumbosacral spine

Common injuries of the thoracolumbar spine include compression fractures, burst fractures, flexion distraction injuries, chance injuries, fracture dislocations, hyperextension injuries, and less significant spinous process and transverse process fractures. The bulk of fractures tend to occur at the thoracolumbar junction between T12 and L2. There are no specific measurements that definitively differentiate stable from unstable injuries.

Historically, it has been suggested that kyphosis greater than 20–30°, height loss greater than 50%, or canal compromise greater than 50% are possible indicators of instability. However, the real predictors of stability for T–L spinal injuries are the integrity of the posterior ligamentous complex and the patient's neurological exam. Certainly, if a patient has greater than 20–30° of focal kyphosis, one must carefully look at the interspinous distance, look for a soft-tissue hematoma, and look at the facet joints for widening indicative of an incompetent ligamentous complex. However, the kyphosis alone is not necessarily indicative of instability. Likewise, 50% height loss may suggest a significant axial load in a young patient but may not be unusual in an elderly osteoporotic individual and hence is not a reliable indicator of instability. With respect to canal compromise, 50% may be significant above the conus where the cord to canal ratio is much lower but may be easily tolerated in the lower lumbar spine. Thus, the degree of canal compromise also does not clearly evaluate instability, but rather it suggests that a more detailed neurological exam is indicated to clearly assess the patient's neurological status. Many of the commonly measured parameters, though helpful in describing an injury, do not help differentiate the stable from the thoracolumbar and lumbosacral injuries.

Extension injuries are unusual in a physiologically healthy individual but are innately unstable injuries in patients with an ankylosing condition, such as ankylosing spondylitis (AS) or diffuse idiopathic skeletal hyperostosis (DISH). Any amount of displacement is suggestive of instability. These are often underappreciated but represent unstable injuries [22].

Summary

There are various radiographic measurements available that are tools in the assessment of spinal trauma, but these must be used appropriately and cautiously with an understanding of their limitations. There are no absolutes and every individual injury has its unique footprint. Although it may be easy to locate and describe fractures, subluxations, and injuries, the fine nuances of stability are much harder to agree on. The advent of CT scans with multiplanar reformats and MRI scans with various sequencing formats has helped greatly in identifying injuries that were previously missed. However, these still rely on interpretation of studies obtained on recumbent patients without exposure to gravitational forces. In addition, while advanced imaging such as CT has undoubtedly enhanced our understanding fracture mechanisms, cumulative radiation exposure from repeated examination and intraoperative imaging may pose significant health risks in the future. Judicious use of costly advanced imaging modalities is recommended. Dynamic x-rays maintain an integral part of radiographic assessment and measurement of trauma patients with unclear structural integrity of their spinal column. Spinal stability is relative and the patient's physiology and expectations must weigh into the appropriate management for each patient. What is considered an acceptable outcome?

5   Radiographic measurements

5.2   Diseases

Introduction

One of the greatest challenges in spine care is the correlation of clinical presentation to structural findings seen on radiographic imaging. While all surgical decisions are based upon clinical and radiographic presentation, the influence of imaging on surgical decision making varies greatly based on the etiology of disease. In spinal deformity and trauma, there exist specific radiographic criteria and thresholds, which guide surgical decision making. Surgery for scoliosis is often recommended based on radiographic imaging in patients without significant symptoms. Conversely, in spinal tumor disease and infection there is a dearth of reliable, reproducible radiographic measures, and much of the radiographic assessment is descriptive. The decision to undergo surgery in these cases is less reliant upon specific imaging measurements.

In some cases, as in degenerative disc disease for instance, radiographic imaging may overestimate spinal pathology. There is a high prevalence of structural abnormalities in asymptomatic patients [1]. The presence of these radiographic abnormali-

ties can often influence diagnosis and subsequent treatments. In this chapter, the authors will illustrate the difficulty in defining certain spinal pathologies by relying on radiographic measures alone. While the correlation of radiographic findings will always need to be correlated with clinical presentation, further investigation into radiographic metrics may help standardize assessment and disease categorization and thus help in developing surgical treatment protocols for the spine.

Evaluation of symptomatic degeneration of the spine

The treatment of degenerative disorders of the spine is commonly based on subjective symptoms (pain and activity limitation), physical examination, and imaging. The assumption that there is little or no correlation between the physical exam and x-rays has led physicians to use imaging studies to assist in their decision making process. Consequently, data regarding measurements of degeneration are rarely present in the literature. Even when reviewing advanced imaging studies, data can be subjective and examiner-dependent. Commonly used metrics usually refer to stability concepts derived from spinal trauma, and therefore may be of limited value in the assessment of degenerative spinal conditions. Descriptions of segmental stability, vertical or axial instability are not supported consistently, thus limiting the comparison of both epidemiological and clinical data.

For degenerative spinal diseases the use of MRI has found increasing popularity in an attempt to "quantify" the magnitude of the disease state, however, with little or no correlation to patients' symptoms. With such uncertainty of foundation, attempts at correlating treatment results with diagnosis becomes a notoriously imprecise undertaking.

Cervical spine

As elsewhere in the spine, presence of imaging abnormalities in the cervical spine should be correlated to the affected patient's clinical presentation. Radiographic measurement of cervical spine pathology has been extensively reported, however the utility of these measurements in clinical decision making varies depending on the etiology of disease.

In patients presenting with axial neck pain, the authors continue to support plain x-rays as arguably the single most useful investigation exam. Plain x-rays can illustrate general alignment and directly reveal atlantoaxial and subaxial instability as well as longstanding degenerative changes. In patients without neurological symptoms in absence of trauma, CT and MRI scans are generally not of great use in defining the primary cause of pain and guiding initial management.

Specific radiographic measures of the cervical spine, such as spinal canal diameter, might lead the physician towards the suspicion of spinal stenosis. While thresholds of canal dimensions have been described, clinicians prefer to describe the appearance of the cervical spine qualitatively rather than with actual quantitative measurements. Neuroimaging with its presence or absence of cerebrospinal fluid anterior or posterior to the cord, myelomalacia, or cord deformation often allow clinicians to express the severity of stenosis and resultant myelopathy directly rather than resorting to normative values.

Spondylotic changes found in x-rays are the result of progressive subluxation of the apophyseal joints due to degenerative changes in facet joints and discs [2–4]. Several authors have attempted to grade the severity of such changes, but in general have failed in correlating clinical presentation and radiographic findings.

Lumbar spine

Degenerative processes can also change the sagittal balance of the spinal column. This has been associated with a variety of signs and symptoms, such as axial pain, myelopathic symptoms, radicular pain, balance and gait difficulties. Uchida et al [5] demonstrated that kyphotic deformity and mechanical stress play an important role in neurological dysfunction in the cervical degenerated spine.

For the cervical spine, determination of spinal canal size may indeed play a very important role in paralysis risk assessment for at-risk patients, while calculation of postural alignment may become more meaningful for identification of neck pain.

The lumbar spine is particularly affected by degenerative changes because of its location, structure, and function. The whole body weight passes through the lumbar spine and the combination of axial and shearing (sagittal) forces puts this region in constant stress. The morphology of intervertebral disc and facet degeneration of the lumbar spine has been frequently described [6–14]. Several grading systems for these degenerative changes have been described. These grading systems invariably rely on qualitative interpretations rather than more objective quantitative measurements. The utility of these grading systems for lumbar disc disease have also not been shown to correlate with guidance of clinical decision making.

Just as with the cervical spine, a number of normative values to quantify lumbar stenosis and spondylolisthesis does exist. However, in clinical reality clinicians seem to strongly prefer qualitative expressions rather than actual measurements. As is the case with the cervical spine, any findings on imaging should be correlated with clinical presentation. In the near future, technological advances and mapping software may allow for more accurate expression of spinal canal compression and vertebral body alignment. This may offer a greater chance of correlating symptoms to imaging findings and eventual treatment outcomes.

Deformity

The Cobb angle is universally utilized in measuring coronal and sagittal spinal deformity. In spinal deformity surgery, radiographic measurements are of eminent importance in assessing severity of disease, likelihood of progression, and surgical planning. In some patients, the radiographic measurement may be the most influential factor in selecting treatment. For example, surgery is often recommended for progressive adolescent idiopathic scoliosis, even if there is minimal pain and dysfunction.

Other metrics of deformity have also proven useful in assessing severity and surgical planning. These include sagittal balance, C7 plumb line, slip angle, and pelvic incidence.

Imaging of spine tumors

Radiographic assessment of spinal tumors is essential in diagnosis and decision making for treatment. Measurement of tumor dimensions, destruction of bone elements of the spinal column (vertebral body, rib heads, facet joints, posterior arches, and pars), osteolytic versus blastic disease, and encroachment into the spinal canal are all important considerations that factor into clinical decision making. While plain imaging remains important, advanced imaging is strongly suggested for comprehensive disease state understanding. CT scans allow for assessment of mineralization of the mass and determination of osteolysis of the spinal column. MRI allows for assessment of soft tissue and neurocompressive pathology. Taneichi et al [15] identified risk factors and the probability of vertebral body collapse in metastasis of the thoracic and lumbar spine based on MRI measurements.

Several classifications and surgical guidelines have considered lesion size. However, these tend to focus on relative size rather than absolute size (dimensions as a percentage of the vertebral body or other adjacent structures). Recently, an effort by the Spine Oncology Study Group has led to new treatment guidelines, where the concept of tumor instability is differentiated from traumatic instability [16]. Percentage of bone involvement and collapse are part of a treatment algorithm that aims to direct surgeons toward the need for instrumentation of tumors. While these are useful, the authors feel that criteria examining absolute measurements would be a helpful addition to further assess the severity of disease. Determination of segmental disease severity should be possible in the near future using mapping software. This could be a valuable aid in research as well as clinical decision making.

Imaging of infections

Infection of the spinal column, similar to tumor disease, lacks specific radiographic standards to assess the severity and provide guidelines for treatment. The radiographic findings that guide decision making include the extent of canal encroachment and neurocompressive pathology, resultant deformity, instability, size and location of abscess formation, and presence of a host response. Akin to management of spinal column tumor disease, preoperative planning for the treatment of infection is best done with CT and/or MRI.

Summary

In our attempts to become more systematic in our management of spinal disorders, important disease categories such as degenerative, neoplastic, and infectious disorders are analyzed with more anecdotally derived quantitative methods, rather than using qualitative criteria. Despite dramatic advances in software resources, which would allow for determination of reasonably precise measurements in affected areas of the spinal column, actual applications of these resources for clinical and even for research purposes have remained uncommon. With the rapidly expanding capacities of databases, improved quantification of disease states should become possible. Availability of such data repositories may enable creation of more meaningful normative values, possibly drive the evolution of clinical decision making tools, and eventually allow for correlation of outcomes with disease states. Especially in the arena of degenerative diseases, attempts at developing objective assessment tools to correlate with outcomes of treatments cannot come too soon.

References

1. **Boden SD, Davis DO, Dina TS, et al** (1990) Abnormal magnetic-resonance scans of the lumbar spine in asymptomatic subjects. A prospective investigation. *J Bone Joint Surg Am;* 72:403–408.

2. **Rao RD, Currier BL, Albert TJ, et al** (2007) Degenerative cervical spondylosis: clinical syndromes, pathogenesis, and management. *J Bone Joint Surg Am;* 89:1360–1378.

3. **Wang B, Liu H, Wang H, et al** (2006) Segmental instability in cervical spondylotic myelopathy with severe disc degeneration. *Spine;* 31:1327–1331.

4. **Zdeblick TA, Bohlman HH** (1989) Cervical kyphosis and myelopathy. Treatment by anterior corpectomy and strut-grafting. *J Bone Joint Surg Am;* 71:170–182.

5. **Uchida K, Nakajima H, Sato R, et al** (2009) Cervical spondylotic myelopathy associated with kyphosis or sagittal sigmoid alignment: outcome after anterior or posterior decompression. *J Neurosurg Spine;* 11:521–528.

6. **Adams MA, Dolan P, Hutton WC** (1986) The stages of disc degeneration as revealed by discograms. *J Bone Joint Surg Br;* 68:36–41.

7. **Collins DH** (1949) *The pathology of articular and spinal diseases.* Edward Arnold & Co: London.

8. **Coventry MB** (1945) The intervertebral disc: its macroscopic anatomy and pathology: Part III. Pathological changes in the intervertebral disc lesion. *J Bone Joint Surg (Am)* 27:460–473.

9. **Coventry MB** (1945) The intervertebral disc: its microscopic anatomy and pathology: Part II. Changes in the intervertebral disc concomitant with age. *J Bone Joint Surg (Am);* 27:233–247.

10. **Friberg S, Hirsch C** (1949) Anatomical and clinical studies on lumbar disc degeneration. *Acta Orthop Scand;* 19:222–242.

11. **Hirsch C** (1971) Some morphological changes in the cervical spine during ageing. *Hirsch C, Zotterman Y (ed), Cervical pain.* Pergamon Press: Oxford, 21–32.

12. **Resnick D** (1985) Degenerative diseases of the vertebral column. *Radiology;* 156:3–14.

13. **Tondury G** (1971) The behaviour of the cervical discs during life. *Hirsch C, Zotterman Y (ed), Cervical pain.* Pergamon Press: Oxford, 59–66.

14. **Vernon-Roberts B, Pirie CJ** (1977) Degenerative changes in the intervertebral discs of the lumbar spine and their sequelae. *Rheumatol Rehabil;* 16:13–21.

15. **Taneichi H, Kaneda K, Takeda N, et al** (1997) Risk factors and probability of vertebral body collapse in metastases of the thoracic and lumbar spine. *Spine;* 22:239–245.

16. **Chan P, Boriani S, Fourney DR, et al** (2009) An assessment of the reliability of the Enneking and Weinstein-Boriani-Biagini classifications for staging of primary spinal tumors by the Spine Oncology Study Group. *Spine;* 34:384–391.

5.2.1   Cervical spine alignment

1   Sagittal alignment

Description
Measured from the superior end plate of C3 to the inferior end plate of C7 on a lateral x-ray.

Interpretation
30–45° of lordosis is the "normal" range, which varies by individual.

Clinical relevance
This measurement indicates the sagittal balance of the cervical spine.

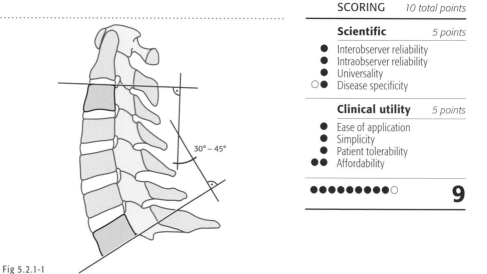

Fig 5.2.1-1

SCORING   *10 total points*

Scientific   *5 points*
- ● Interobserver reliability
- ● Intraobserver reliability
- ●● Universality
- ○● Disease specificity

Clinical utility   *5 points*
- ● Ease of application
- ● Simplicity
- ● Patient tolerability
- ●● Affordability

●●●●●●●●●○   **9**

Reliability

Population tested in	Interobserver reliability	Intraobserver reliability
X-rays of volunteers (N = 30) were measured twice by two orthopaedic surgeons to determine cervical total and segmental sagittal angular values [1]	+	+

References:
1. Hardacker JW, Shuford RF, Capicotto PN, et al (1997) Radiographic standing cervical segmental alignment in adult volunteers without neck symptoms. *Spine (Phila Pa 1976)*; discussion 1480.

2   Coronal alignment

Description

Normal coronal alignment is zero;
specifically C7 is centered over the
pelvis on a standing x-ray.

On a standing full length x-ray, the C7
plumb line should fall within a few
millimeters of the center of the
sacrum, and should be colinear with
the central sacral vertical line (CSVL).

Interpretation

0° of deviation on the coronal plane is
the norm.

Clinical relevance

This measurement indicates the
coronal balance of the cervical spine.

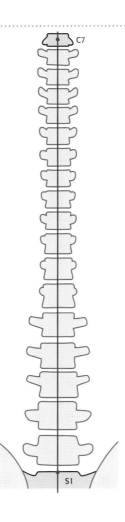

Fig 5.2.1-2

SCORING   *10 total points*

Scientific   *5 points*

○   Interobserver reliability
○   Intraobserver reliability
●   Universality
○● Disease specificity

Clinical utility   *5 points*

●   Ease of application
●   Simplicity
●   Patient tolerability
●● Affordability

●●●●●●●○○○   **7**

Reliability

Population tested in	Interobserver reliability	Intraobserver reliability
Not tested		

3   Lordotic alignment

SCORING   *10 total points*

Description

The distance between the center of the cervical curve and the line connecting the posterior edge of the odontoid process and the posteroinferior edge of the 7th vertebral body.

Interpretation

Distance ≥ 2 mm is defined as lordotic alignment.

Clinical relevance

This measurement indicates the sagittal balance of the cervical spine.

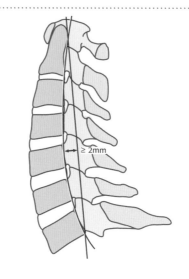

Fig 5.2.1-3

Scientific   *5 points*

○ Interobserver reliability
○ Intraobserver reliability
● Universality
○● Disease specificity

Clinical utility   *5 points*

● Ease of application
● Simplicity
● Patient tolerability
●● Affordability

●●●●●●●○○○   **7**

Reliability

Population tested in	Interobserver reliability	Intraobserver reliability
Not tested		

5.2.2   Cervical spine degenerative measurements

1   Pavlov-Torg index [1] (cervical stenosis)

Description
The sagittal diameter of the spinal canal is measured from the posterior aspect of the midvertebral body to the spinolaminar line in a lateral x-ray image. A spinal canal (A) to vertebral body sagittal diameter (B) ratio is calculated.

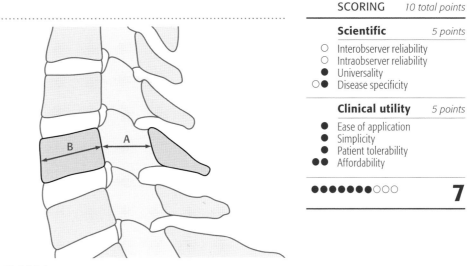

Interpretation
14–22 mm represents the normal range of the sagittal diameter of the spinal canal as measured on a lateral C-spine x-ray.

Pavlov-Torg ratio: A/B

Fig 5.2.2-1

If = 1.0 then it is normal.
If ≤ 0.8 then it is stenotic.
If 0.8 or less then it correlates with an increased risk of developing myelopathy.

Reliability

Population tested in	Interobserver reliability	Intraobserver reliability
Not tested		

Clinical relevance
A ratio of 0.8 or less as seen on lateral x-rays with clinical correlation suggests that advanced imaging is warranted to examine the spinal canal and cord in more detail.

References:
1. Pavlov H, Torg JS, Robie B, et al (1987) Cervical spinal stenosis: determination with vertebral body ratio method. *Radiology;* 164:771-775.

2   Spinal stenosis (MRI measurements)

Description
Measurements of the cross-sectional area of the dural sac.

Interpretation
Qualitative (degree of stenosis):
Mild: ≤1/3 of its normal size
Moderate: between 1/3 and 2/3 of
          normal size
Severe: >2/3 of normal size

Quantitative:
Measurements included cross-sectional areas of the osseous spinal canal, the soft tissue spinal canal, and thecal sac area. Spinal canal and thecal sac area were measured both at the level of the disc and, when possible, at the pedicle level above. This allowed for calculation of the stenosis ratio obtained by dividing the thecal sac area at the disc level by the area at the pedicle level.

Clinical relevance
Though more expensive, the MRI allows for a qualitative and quantitative assessment of the spinal canal and possible cord compression. MRI has become the standard for advanced imaging of the spine.

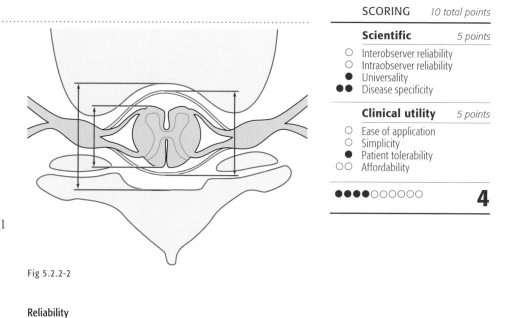

Fig 5.2.2-2

SCORING   10 total points

Scientific   5 points
○ Interobserver reliability
○ Intraobserver reliability
● Universality
●● Disease specificity

Clinical utility   5 points
○ Ease of application
○ Simplicity
● Patient tolerability
○○ Affordability

●●●●○○○○○○   **4**

Reliability

Population tested in	Interobserver reliability	Intraobserver reliability
Not tested		

3 Sagittal diameter of the spinal canal

Description
Measured from the posterior aspect of the midvertebral body to the spinolaminar line in a lateral x-ray image.

Interpretation
14–22 mm represents the normal range of the mid-sagittal diameter of the spinal canal.

The sagittal diameter of the spinal canal < 13 mm is considered stenotic, and it can predispose to a cervical myelopathy.

≤ 12 mm: relative stenosis

< 9 mm: absolute stenosis

Clinical relevance
This measurement indicates the severity of the bony stenosis as seen on a lateral C-spine x-ray. If clinically correlated, advanced imaging to further evaluate may be indicated.

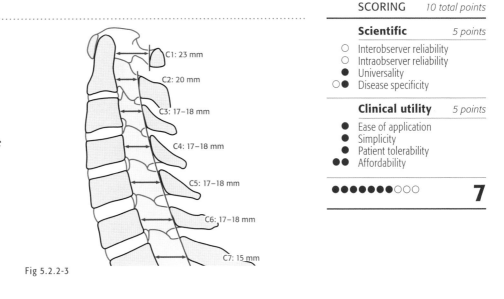

C1: 23 mm
C2: 20 mm
C3: 17–18 mm
C4: 17–18 mm
C5: 17–18 mm
C6: 17–18 mm
C7: 15 mm

Fig 5.2.2-3

Reliability

Population tested in	Interobserver reliability	Intraobserver reliability
Not tested		

4   Interfacet distance (coronal diameter)

SCORING   *10 total points*

Description
Measured in the coronal view and from the medial right facet border to the medial left facet border in an AP x-ray image or axial MRI image.

Interpretation
Average distance: 13 mm

These distances are relatively constant between levels, with individual variations ranging from 9–16 mm.

Clinical relevance
Substantial disparity in measurements between adjacent levels may suggest structural pathology, such as trauma or neoplasm.

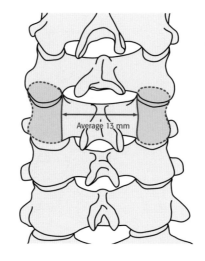

Average 13 mm

Fig 5.2.2-4

Scientific	5 points
○ Interobserver reliability	
○ Intraobserver reliability	
● Universality	
○● Disease specificity	

Clinical utility	5 points
● Ease of application	
● Simplicity	
● Patient tolerability	
○● Affordability	

●●●●●●○○○○   **6**

Reliability

Population tested in	Interobserver reliability	Intraobserver reliability
Not tested		

5   Transverse diameter of the spinal cord

Description
Measured in the axial incidence on
MRI.

Interpretation
Maximal transverse diameter:
13–14 mm

Maximal transverse areas:
- 85.8 + 7.2 mm² at C4-5
- 58.3 + 6.7 mm² at C6

There is, however, considerable
variation in size of the spinal cord due
to the increased nerve supply to upper
limbs. The cervical cord enlarges from
C3 and becomes maximal at C6.

Clinical relevance
Decreased diameter of the spinal cord
may be secondary to neurological
disease, atrophy, or external
compression and, if clinically
correlated, may warrant interventional
treatment.

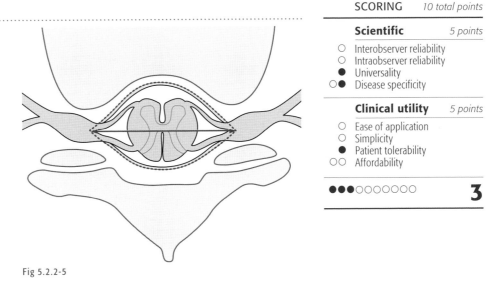

Fig 5.2.2-5

SCORING   *10 total points*

Scientific   *5 points*
○ Interobserver reliability
○ Intraobserver reliability
● Universality
○● Disease specificity

Clinical utility   *5 points*
○ Ease of application
○ Simplicity
● Patient tolerability
○○ Affordability

●●●○○○○○○○   **3**

Reliability

Population tested in	Interobserver reliability	Intraobserver reliability
Not tested		

6   Vertical diameter of the foramen

Description
Measured from the inferior aspect of
the superior articular pilar to the
superior aspect of the inferior articular
pilar.

Interpretation
Ranges from 4–6 mm.

Clinical relevance
As asymptomatic foraminal stenosis
may be fairly prevalent, this
radiographic finding should be
correlated clinically prior to
considering interventional treatment.

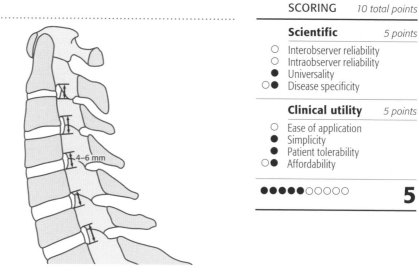

Fig 5.2.2-6

SCORING   *10 total points*

Scientific   *5 points*
○   Interobserver reliability
○   Intraobserver reliability
●   Universality
○● Disease specificity

Clinical utility   *5 points*
○   Ease of application
●   Simplicity
●   Patient tolerability
○● Affordability

●●●●●○○○○○   **5**

Reliability

Population tested in	Interobserver reliability	Intraobserver reliability
Not tested		

7   Horizontal diameter of the foramen

Description
Measured from the posterior aspect of the uncinate process to the anterior aspect of the superior articular process.

Interpretation
Normal value approximately 4 mm.

Clinical relevance
As asymptomatic foraminal stenosis may be fairly prevalent, this radiographic finding should be correlated clinically prior to considering interventional treatment.

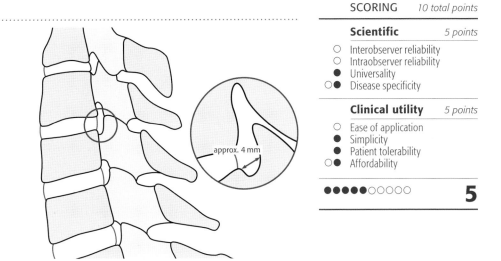

approx. 4 mm

Fig 5.2.2-7

SCORING   *10 total points*

Scientific   *5 points*
○ Interobserver reliability
○ Intraobserver reliability
● Universality
○● Disease specificity

Clinical utility   *5 points*
○ Ease of application
● Simplicity
● Patient tolerability
○● Affordability

●●●●●○○○○○   **5**

Reliability

Population tested in	Interobserver reliability	Intraobserver reliability
Not tested		

8   Foramina exit angle

Description
Measured in the midsagittal plane.

Interpretation
Normal average range: 45°

Clinical relevance
Questionable clinical relevance as
there may be substantial variability
from patient to patient. Generally, this
measurement is not utilized commonly
in clinical decision making.

SCORING   *10 total points*

Scientific   *5 points*

○   Interobserver reliability
○   Intraobserver reliability
●   Universality
○○ Disease specificity

Clinical utility   *5 points*

○   Ease of application
●   Simplicity
●   Patient tolerability
○● Affordability

●●●●○○○○○○   **4**

Illustration not provided as it is not possible to see the nerve root
of the foramen on a midsagittal view.

Reliability

Population tested in	Interobserver reliability	Intraobserver reliability
Not tested		

9   Disc height (normal values)

Description
Anterior disc height divided by the AP diameter of the cranial vertebral body multiplied by 100.

Interpretation
Normal values of anterior disc height normalized to the AP diameter of the cranial vertebral body (=100%).

C2/3: approximately 34%
C3/4: approximately 38%
C4/5: approximately 39%
C5/6: approximately 38%
C6/7: approximately 34%

Clinical relevance
Radiographic disc heights loosely reflect the progression of degenerative disc disease and cervical spondylosis. While decreased disc height does correlate with the vertical diameter of the foramen, correlation with clinical presentation is necessary before treatment or additional imaging studies.

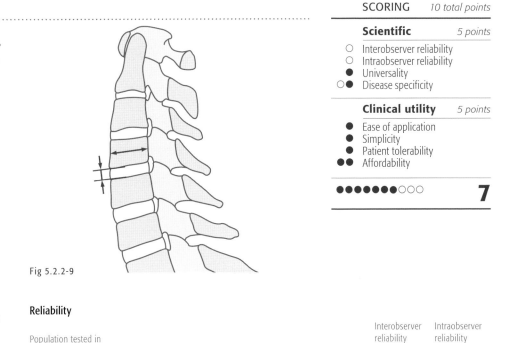

Fig 5.2.2-9

SCORING	10 total points
Scientific	5 points

○ Interobserver reliability
○ Intraobserver reliability
● Universality
○● Disease specificity

Clinical utility	5 points

● Ease of application
● Simplicity
● Patient tolerability
●● Affordability

●●●●●●●○○○   **7**

Reliability

Population tested in	Interobserver reliability	Intraobserver reliability
Not tested		

10   Disc height (degenerated)

Description
The anterior and posterior edges of the adjacent vertebral bodies are defined as those points having the largest distance to the center of the vertebral body. Then, the distance of each of these four edges to the midplane of the disc is measured.

Interpretation
Disc height, osteophyte formation, and diffuse sclerosis make up the overall degree of degeneration of a new radiographic grading system for intervertebral disc degeneration.

The sum of the two anterior distances is defined as actual anterior disc height, and the sum of the two posterior distances is defined as actual posterior disc height.

This actual height is compared to the respective height before degeneration, which is estimated based on the normal values.

Clinical relevance
The radiographic disc heights loosely reflect the progression of degenerative disc disease and cervical spondylosis. While decreased disc height does correlate with the vertical diameter of the foramen, correlation with clinical presentation is necessary before treatment or additional imaging studies.

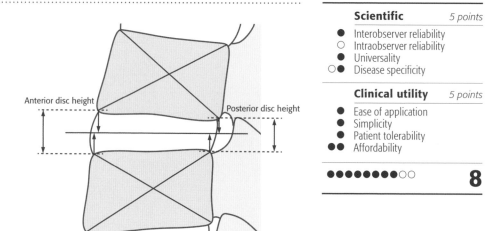

Fig 5.2.2-10

SCORING   *10 total points*

Scientific   *5 points*
● Interobserver reliability
○ Intraobserver reliability
● Universality
○● Disease specificity

Clinical utility   *5 points*
● Ease of application
● Simplicity
● Patient tolerability
●● Affordability

●●●●●●●●○○   **8**

Reliability

Population tested in	Interobserver reliability	Intraobserver reliability
Cervical spinal x-rays of patients (N = 57) evaluated by one experienced observer and one inexperienced observer [1]	+	NA

References:
1. Kettler A, Rohlmann F, Neidlinger-Wilke C, et al (2006) Validity and interobserver agreement of a new radiographic grading system for intervertebral disc degeneration: Part II. Cervical spine. *Eur Spine J;* 15:732-741.

11   Osteophyte formation

Description
The number of osteophytes found in the sagittal x-ray view is counted and their length is measured.

The four AP edges of the adjacent vertebral bodies are evaluated.

Interpretation
Disc height, osteophyte formation, and diffuse sclerosis make up the overall degree of degeneration of a new radiographic grading system for intervertebral disc degeneration.

The sum of the heights of the four osteophytes.

Clinical relevance
Nonspecific osteophytosis generally indicates degenerative changes within the spinal column.

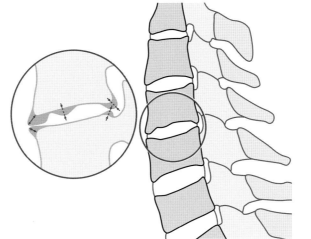

Fig 5.2.2-11

SCORING	10 total points

Scientific	5 points
● Interobserver reliability	
○ Intraobserver reliability	
● Universality	
○● Disease specificity	

Clinical utility	5 points
○ Ease of application	
● Simplicity	
● Patient tolerability	
●● Affordability	

●●●●●●●○○○   **7**

Reliability

Population tested in	Interobserver reliability	Intraobserver reliability
Cervical spinal x-rays of patients (N = 57) evaluated by one experienced observer and one inexperienced observer [1]	+	NA

References:
1. Kettler A, Rohlmann F, Neidlinger-Wilke C, et al (2006) Validity and interobserver agreement of a new radiographic grading system for intervertebral disc degeneration: Part II. Cervical spine. *Eur Spine J;* 15:732-741.

12   Diffuse sclerosis

Description
The lower half of the upper vertebral body and the upper half of the lower vertebral body are each divided into two regions.

Interpretation
Disc height, osteophyte formation, and diffuse sclerosis make up the overall degree of degeneration of a new radiographic grading system for intervertebral disc degeneration.

The number of regions covered by sclerosis is counted.

A partially covered region is counted as if it was completely covered.

Clinical relevance
Though often noted on radiographic review, this is generally a nonspecific finding and correlation with clinical presentation and other radiographic features are recommended.

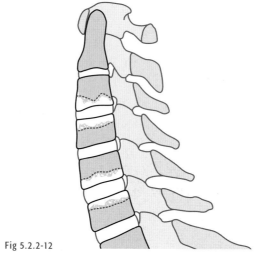

Fig 5.2.2-12

SCORING	10 total points
Scientific	5 points

● Interobserver reliability
○ Intraobserver reliability
○ Universality
○● Disease specificity

Clinical utility	5 points

● Ease of application
○ Simplicity
● Patient tolerability
●● Affordability

●●●●●●○○○○   **6**

Reliability

Population tested in	Interobserver reliability	Intraobserver reliability
Cervical spinal x-rays of patients (N = 57) evaluated by one experienced observer and one inexperienced observer [1]	+	NA

References:
1. Kettler A, Rohlmann F, Neidlinger-Wilke C, et al (2006) Validity and interobserver agreement of a new radiographic grading system for intervertebral disc degeneration: Part II. Cervical spine. *Eur Spine J;* 15:732-741.

5.2.3   Cervical spine in kyphosis and segmental instability associated with cervical spondylotic myelopathy

1   Kyphotic angle

Description

Measured on lateral x-rays obtained in the neutral and flexion positions between the two lines at the posterior margin of the most cranial and caudal vertebral bodies forming maximal kyphosis through C2 to C7.

Interpretation

Normal cervical spine alignment in the sagittal plane is in lordosis, and a kyphosis angle higher than 10° is associated with a higher chance of cervical myelopathy.

Clinical relevance

Severe kyphosis can be symptomatic and may require surgical treatment. When combined with myelopathy, this finding can heavily influence the surgical approach and strategy.

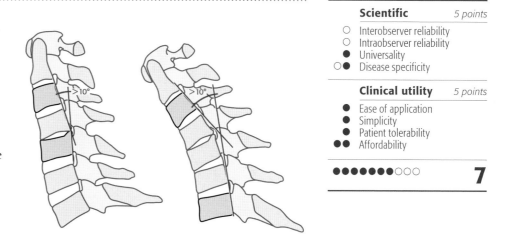

Fig 5.2.3-1

SCORING	10 total points
Scientific	5 points

○ Interobserver reliability
○ Intraobserver reliability
● Universality
○● Disease specificity

Clinical utility	5 points

● Ease of application
● Simplicity
● Patient tolerability
●● Affordability

●●●●●●●○○○   **7**

Reliability

Population tested in	Interobserver reliability	Intraobserver reliability
Not tested		

2   Anterior spondylolisthesis

Description
The distance between the posteroinferior edge of the superior vertebral body and the posterosuperior edge of the inferior vertebral body.

Interpretation
Anterior vertebral translation > 3 mm in the sagittal plane suggests spondylolisthesis.

Clinical relevance
It is often associated with neck pain and spinal stenosis.

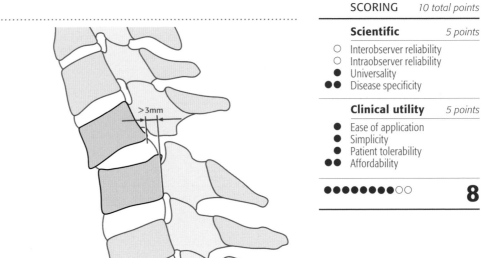

Fig 5.2.3-2

Scientific   *5 points*

○ Interobserver reliability
○ Intraobserver reliability
● Universality
●● Disease specificity

Clinical utility   *5 points*

● Ease of application
● Simplicity
● Patient tolerability
●● Affordability

●●●●●●●●○○   **8**

Reliability

Population tested in	Interobserver reliability	Intraobserver reliability
Not tested		

3   Vertebral slip angle

Description
The angle obtained between the inferior vertebral plate of the superior vertebra and a line drawn parallel to the superior vertebral plate of the inferior vertebra in the sagittal plane.

Interpretation
Anterior rotation > 10° in the sagittal plane suggests a vertebral slip.

Clinical relevance
This measurement additionally indicates sagittal plane deformity of the cervical spine.

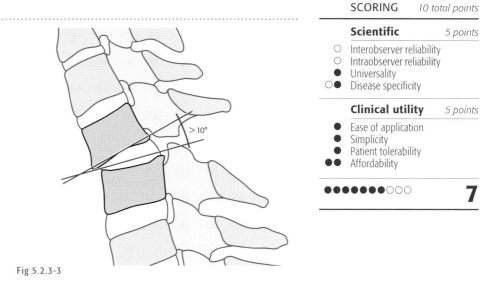

Fig 5.2.3-3

SCORING   *10 total points*

Scientific   *5 points*

○ Interobserver reliability
○ Intraobserver reliability
● Universality
○● Disease specificity

Clinical utility   *5 points*

● Ease of application
● Simplicity
● Patient tolerability
●● Affordability

●●●●●●●○○○   **7**

Reliability

Population tested in	Interobserver reliability	Intraobserver reliability
Not tested		

4   Reversed dynamic spinal canal stenosis

Description
The distance between the posterior superior edge of the vertebral body and the anterior edge of the lamina one segment above.

Interpretation
In the flexion position ≤ 12 mm on a flexion x-ray suggests reversed dynamic spinal canal stenosis.

Clinical relevance
This measurement indicates the severity of the bony stenosis as seen on a lateral C-spine x-ray. If clinically correlated, advanced imaging to further evaluate may be indicated.

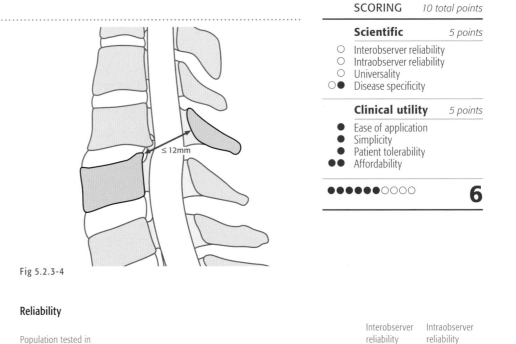

Fig 5.2.3-4

SCORING   *10 total points*

Scientific   *5 points*
○ Interobserver reliability
○ Intraobserver reliability
○ Universality
○● Disease specificity

Clinical utility   *5 points*
● Ease of application
● Simplicity
● Patient tolerability
●● Affordability

●●●●●●○○○○   **6**

Reliability

Population tested in	Interobserver reliability	Intraobserver reliability
Not tested		

5.2.4 Cervical range of motion

1 Flexion and extension

Description
Movement in the sagittal plane.

Interpretation
Normal range of motion:
approximately 140°

Clinical relevance
The overall tendency is that range of motion varies among individuals and decreases as age increases. Attention should be given to changes in serial exams or asymmetry.

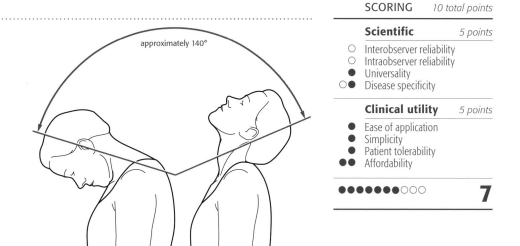

approximately 140°

Fig 5.2.4-1

Reliability

Population tested in	Interobserver reliability	Intraobserver reliability
Not tested		

2   Lateral bending

Description
Movement in the coronal plane.

Interpretation
Normal range of motion:
approximately 90°

Clinical relevance
The overall tendency is that range of
motion varies among individuals and
decreases as age increases. Attention
should be given to changes in serial
exams or asymmetry.

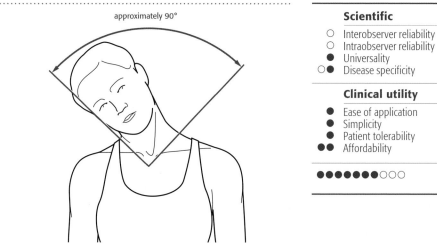

approximately 90°

Fig 5.2.4-2

SCORING   *10 total points*

Scientific   *5 points*
○ Interobserver reliability
○ Intraobserver reliability
● Universality
○● Disease specificity

Clinical utility   *5 points*
● Ease of application
● Simplicity
● Patient tolerability
●● Affordability

●●●●●●●○○○   **7**

Reliability

Population tested in	Interobserver reliability	Intraobserver reliability
Not tested		

3   Axial rotation

Description
Rotation of the head with a neutral cervical spine.

Interpretation
Normal range of motion: approximately 175°

Clinical relevance
The overall tendency is that range of motion varies among individuals and decreases as age increases. Attention should be given to changes in serial exams or asymmetry.

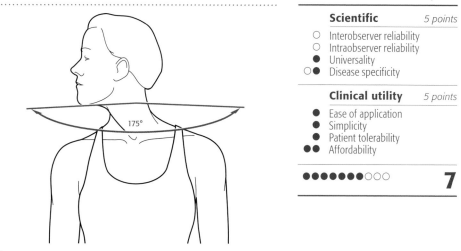

Fig 5.2.4-3

SCORING   *10 total points*

Scientific   *5 points*
- ○ Interobserver reliability
- ○ Intraobserver reliability
- ● Universality
- ○● Disease specificity

Clinical utility   *5 points*
- ● Ease of application
- ● Simplicity
- ● Patient tolerability
- ●● Affordability

●●●●●●○○○   **7**

Reliability

Population tested in	Interobserver reliability	Intraobserver reliability
Not tested		

4   Rotation from flexion

Description
Rotation of the head with a flexed cervical spine.

Interpretation
Normal range of motion: approximately 80°

Clinical relevance
The overall tendency is that range of motion varies among individuals and decreases as age increases. Attention should be given to changes in serial exams or asymmetry.

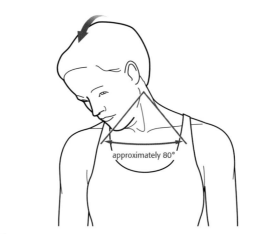

approximately 80°

Fig 5.2.4-4

SCORING   *10 total points*

Scientific   *5 points*
- ○ Interobserver reliability
- ○ Intraobserver reliability
- ● Universality
- ○● Disease specificity

Clinical utility   *5 points*
- ● Ease of application
- ● Simplicity
- ● Patient tolerability
- ●● Affordability

●●●●●●●○○○   **7**

Reliability

Population tested in	Interobserver reliability	Intraobserver reliability
Not tested		

5   Rotation from extension

Description
Rotation of the head with an extended cervical spine.

Interpretation
Normal range of motion: approximately 165°

Clinical relevance
The overall tendency is that range of motion varies among individuals and decreases as age increases. Attention should be given to changes in serial exams or asymmetry.

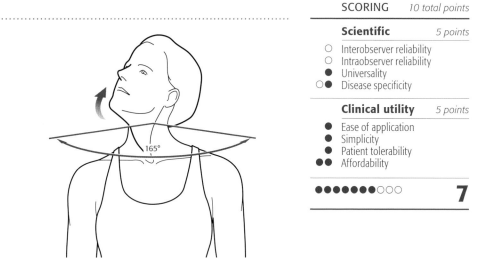

Fig 5.2.4-5

SCORING   *10 total points*

Scientific	*5 points*
○	Interobserver reliability
○	Intraobserver reliability
●	Universality
○●	Disease specificity

Clinical utility	*5 points*
●	Ease of application
●	Simplicity
●	Patient tolerability
●●	Affordability

●●●●●●●○○○   **7**

Reliability

Population tested in	Interobserver reliability	Intraobserver reliability
Not tested		

5.2.5   Assessment of cervical fusion

1   Manual measurement

Description
Spinous process distance equals the measurement in flexion/magnification factor minus the measurement in extension/magnification factor. The magnification factor equals the measurement of plate length on the x-ray divided by the actual plate length.

The displacement measured between the tips of the spinous processes has been shown to be a better representation of the manual measurement techniques.

Interpretation
Normal: < 1 mm

Clinical relevance
Motion between the spinous processes at a level of fusion indicates a nonbony union of the level.

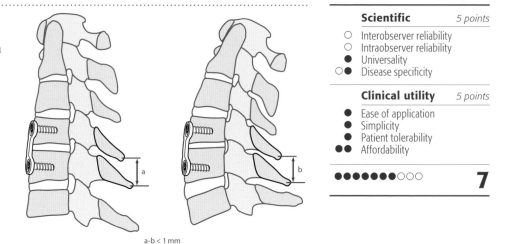

a-b < 1 mm

Fig 5.2.5-1

SCORING   *10 total points*

Scientific   *5 points*

○ Interobserver reliability
○ Intraobserver reliability
● Universality
○● Disease specificity

Clinical utility   *5 points*

● Ease of application
● Simplicity
● Patient tolerability
●● Affordability

●●●●●●●○○○   **7**

Reliability

Population tested in	Interobserver reliability	Intraobserver reliability
Not tested		

2   Quantitative motion analysis (QMA)

Description

The software superimposes the flexion and extension x-rays to determine the angular motion at an intervertebral level.

Uses a QMA software (Medical Metrics, Inc.) that utilizes all of the vertebral surface anatomy available on the lateral radiographic images for tracking and is not affected by the placement of landmarks. Rotations are calculated from the transformation matrices describing the change in position of each vertebra between the flexion and extension images. The software also corrects for differences in magnification between the images.

Interpretation

Normal: < 1.5° of angular motion

Clinical relevance

Though perhaps more accurate in detecting motion at a fusion site, QMA requires software for easy utilization in a clinical setting.

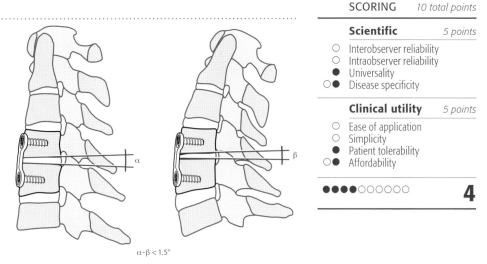

$\alpha - \beta < 1.5°$

Fig 5.2.5-2

Reliability

Population tested in	Interobserver reliability	Intraobserver reliability
Not tested		

SCORING   *10 total points*

Scientific	*5 points*
○ Interobserver reliability	
○ Intraobserver reliability	
● Universality	
○● Disease specificity	

Clinical utility	*5 points*
○ Ease of application	
○ Simplicity	
● Patient tolerability	
○● Affordability	

●●●●○○○○○○   **4**

5.2.6   Motion adjacent to fusion

1   Posteroanterior (dorsoventral) displacement

Description

Distance between the projections of the center points (geometric center of the vertebral body corners) of the vertebrae onto the bisectrix, divided by the mean depth of the cranial vertebra.

Displacement depends linearly on the sagittal plane angle. A correction is applied in order to permit comparisons among x-rays taken in different postures of the cervical spine. Angle-corrected displacement is independent of the posture of the cervical spine adopted when the x-ray was taken.

Interpretation

Positive, if the cranial vertebra is displaced in an anterior direction with respect to the caudal vertebra.

Clinical relevance

Suggestive of advanced degenerative changes, which may be correlated to neurocompressive pathology.

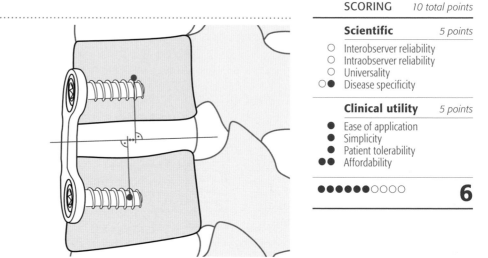

Fig 5.2.6-1

SCORING   *10 total points*

Scientific   *5 points*

○ Interobserver reliability
○ Intraobserver reliability
○ Universality
○● Disease specificity

Clinical utility   *5 points*

● Ease of application
● Simplicity
● Patient tolerability
●● Affordability

●●●●●●○○○○   **6**

Reliability

Population tested in	Interobserver reliability	Intraobserver reliability
Not tested		

2 Sagittal plane rotational motion

Description
Difference between the sagittal plane angle in the extension view minus angle in the flexion view.

Interpretation
If there is substantial disparity between the motion measured at the level adjacent to the fusion as compared to the other unfused levels or an earlier measurement at the same level, this is suggestive of advanced degenerative changes.

Clinical relevance
This hypermobility adjacent to a fusion suggests advanced degenerative changes and may correlate with neurocompressive pathology.

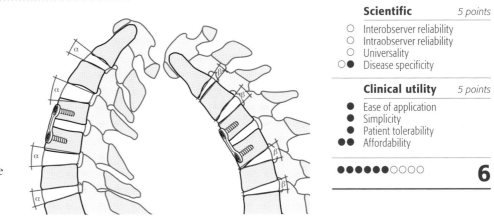

α-β = Sagittal plane rotational motion

Fig 5.2.6-2

Reliability

Population tested in	Interobserver reliability	Intraobserver reliability
Not tested		

3   Sagittal plane translational motion

SCORING   *10 total points*

Description
Difference between the displacement in the extension view minus displacement in the flexion view.

Interpretation
Normal values:
C2/3: -8 to -15%
C3/4: -13 to -29%
C4/5: -12 to -20%
C5/6: -8 to -14%
C6/7: -5 to +5%

The values are calculated in a percentage of the mean depth of the caudal vertebrae.

Clinical relevance
Suggestive of advanced degenerative changes, which may be correlated to neurocompressive pathology.

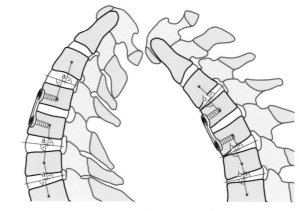

a-b = Sagittal plane translational motion

Fig 5.2.6-3

Scientific   *5 points*
○ Interobserver reliability
○ Intraobserver reliability
○ Universality
○● Disease specificity

Clinical utility   *5 points*
● Ease of application
● Simplicity
● Patient tolerability
●● Affordability

●●●●●●○○○○   **6**

Reliability

Population tested in	Interobserver reliability	Intraobserver reliability
Not tested		

4   Interspinous distance

Description
The difference in the distance of adjacent spinous process tips as measured on flexion and extension views.

Interpretation
More than 2 mm suggests the presence of nonunion.

Clinical relevance
Suggestive of bony nonunion and persistent pathological motion at the measured levels.

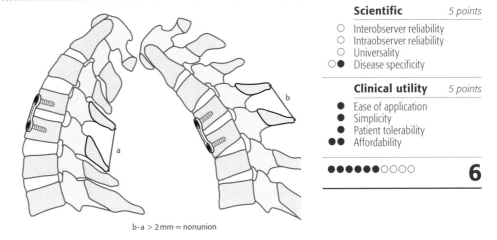

b-a > 2 mm = nonunion

Fig 5.2.6-4

SCORING   *10 total points*

Scientific   *5 points*
- ○ Interobserver reliability
- ○ Intraobserver reliability
- ○ Universality
- ○● Disease specificity

Clinical utility   *5 points*
- ● Ease of application
- ● Simplicity
- ● Patient tolerability
- ●● Affordability

●●●●●●○○○○   **6**

Reliability

Population tested in	Interobserver reliability	Intraobserver reliability
Not tested		

5.2.7   Progression of ossification of the posterior longitudinal ligament (OPLL)

1   Radiographic method

Description

Anchor points (ie, four corners of each vertebral body) are marked on each x-ray, and reference lines (lines that pass the midpoints of the anchor points at both vertebral and intervertebral levels) and reference points (midpoints of anterior anchor points at both vertebral and intervertebral levels) are set based on these anchor points. The distances between these reference lines and points and the upper, lower, and posterior margins of ossified lesions were measured to represent the length and thickness of OPLL.

Interpretation

A criterion of progression was set as a 2 mm increase in the size of an ossified mass in any direction.

Clinical relevance

This method did not gain wide acceptance because it was time consuming and complicated, requiring many lines and points to be drawn.

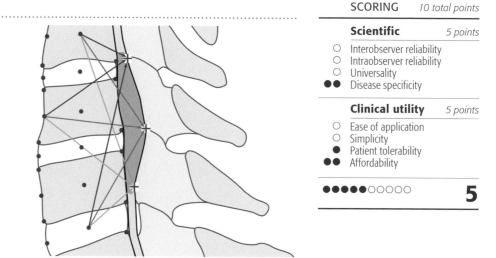

Fig 5.2.7-1

Reliability

Population tested in	Interobserver reliability	Intraobserver reliability
Not tested		

2 Computer-assisted measurement system: length of an ossified lesion

Description
Distances from the marked points at the upper and lower ends of a lesion to the nearest reference lines are measured automatically.

Interpretation
The difference in the values obtained between two time points is defined as progression of ossification in the craniocaudal direction.

Clinical relevance
Yields a more accurate assessment of progression than qualitative analysis. However, this requires computer software and may not necessarily influence clinical decision making.

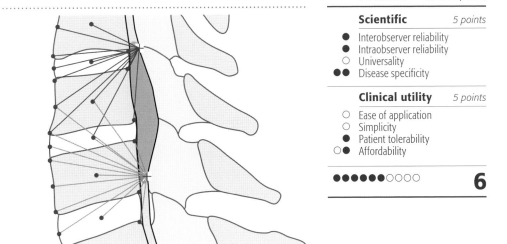

Fig 5.2.7-2

SCORING	10 total points

Scientific	5 points
● Interobserver reliability	
● Intraobserver reliability	
○ Universality	
●● Disease specificity	

Clinical utility	5 points
○ Ease of application	
○ Simplicity	
● Patient tolerability	
○● Affordability	

●●●●●●○○○○   **6**

Reliability

Population tested in	Interobserver reliability	Intraobserver reliability
Lateral cervical x-rays of patients (N = 9) evaluated for length of ossified lesions by eight board-certified spine surgeons [1]	+	+

References:
1. Chiba K, Kato Y, Tsuzuki N, et al (2005) Computer-assisted measurement of the size of ossification in patients with ossification of the posterior longitudinal ligament in the cervical spine. J Orthop Sci; 10:451-456.

3   Computer-assisted measurement system: thickness of an ossified lesion

Description
Distances from the reference points to the points on every reference line that intersects the dorsal margin of the lesion are measured automatically.

Interpretation
The difference in the values obtained between two time points is defined as progression of ossification in the ventrodorsal direction.

Clinical relevance
Yields a more accurate assessment of progression than qualitative analysis, however, this requires computer software and may not necessarily influence clinical decision making.

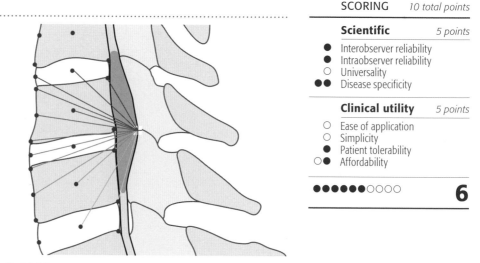

Fig 5.2.7-3

SCORING   *10 total points*

Scientific   *5 points*
● Interobserver reliability
● Intraobserver reliability
○ Universality
●● Disease specificity

Clinical utility   *5 points*
○ Ease of application
○ Simplicity
● Patient tolerability
○● Affordability

●●●●●●○○○○   **6**

Reliability

Population tested in	Interobserver reliability	Intraobserver reliability
Lateral cervical x-rays of patients (N=9) evaluated for thickness of ossified lesions by eight board-certified spine surgeons [1]	+	+

References:
1. Chiba K, Kato Y, Tsuzuki N, et al (2005) Computer-assisted measurement of the size of ossification in patients with ossification of the posterior longitudinal ligament in the cervical spine. *J Orthop Sci;* 10:451-456.

5.2.8   Lumbar spine normal alignment

1   Sagittal alignment

Description
Measured from the superior end plate of T12 to the inferior end plate of S1 on standing x-rays.

Interpretation
Normal range of lumbar lordosis: 40–60°

It can vary between individuals. There is approximately 30° more lordosis than thoracic kyphosis. For a full-length standing x-ray with the knees extended, the C7 plumb line should pass within a few millimeters of the posterior superior corner of S1.

Clinical relevance
This measurement indicates the sagittal balance of the lumbar spine.

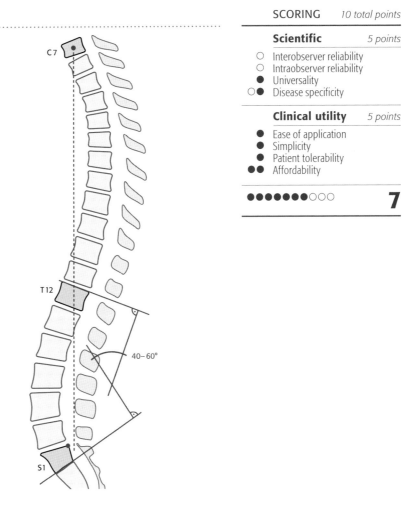

Fig 5.2.8-1

SCORING   *10 total points*

Scientific   *5 points*
○ Interobserver reliability
○ Intraobserver reliability
● Universality
○● Disease specificity

Clinical utility   *5 points*
● Ease of application
● Simplicity
● Patient tolerability
●● Affordability

●●●●●●●○○○   **7**

Reliability

Population tested in	Interobserver reliability	Intraobserver reliability
Not tested		

2   Coronal alignment

Description
Normal coronal alignment is zero; specifically, C7 is centered over the pelvis.

Interpretation
Normal angle: 0°

On a standing full length x-ray, the C7 plumb line should fall within a few millimeters of the center of the sacrum, and should be colinear with the central sacral vertical line (CSVL).

Clinical relevance
This measurement indicates the coronal balance of the lumbar spine.

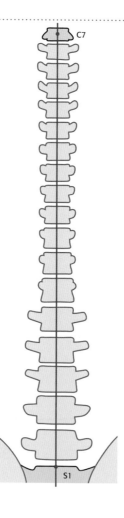

Fig 5.2.8-2

SCORING   *10 total points*

Scientific   *5 points*
- ○ Interobserver reliability
- ○ Intraobserver reliability
- ● Universality
- ○● Disease specificity

Clinical utility   *5 points*
- ● Ease of application
- ● Simplicity
- ● Patient tolerability
- ●● Affordability

●●●●●●●○○○   **7**

Reliability

Population tested in	Interobserver reliability	Intraobserver reliability
Not tested		

5.2.9   Lumbar range of motion

1   Flexion

Description
Movement in the sagittal plane.

Interpretation
Normal range of motion: 40–60°

Clinical relevance
The overall tendency is that range of
motion varies among individuals and
decreases as age increases. Attention
should be given to changes in serial
exams or asymmetry.

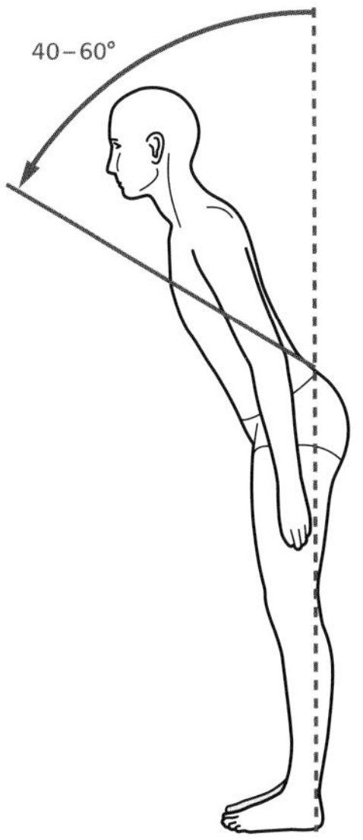

40–60°

Fig 5.2.9-1

SCORING *10 total points*

Scientific *5 points*
- ○ Interobserver reliability
- ○ Intraobserver reliability
- ● Universality
- ○● Disease specificity

Clinical utility *5 points*
- ● Ease of application
- ● Simplicity
- ● Patient tolerability
- ●● Affordability

●●●●●●○○○   **7**

Reliability

Population tested in	Interobserver reliability	Intraobserver reliability
Not tested		

2   Extension

Description
Movement in the sagittal plane.

Interpretation
Normal range of motion: 20–35°

Clinical relevance
The overall tendency is that range of motion varies among individuals and decreases as age increases. Attention should be given to changes in serial exams or asymmetry.

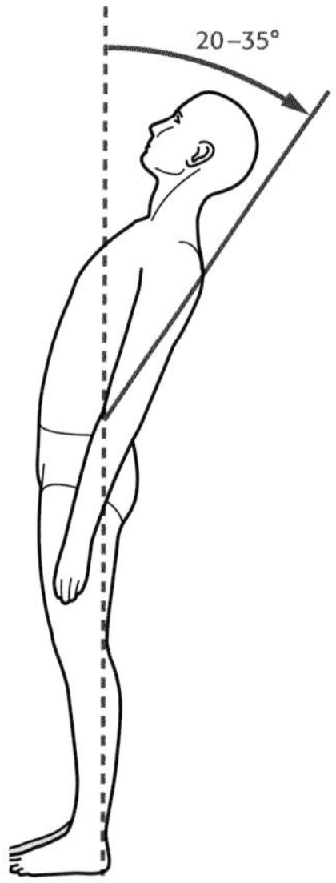

20–35°

Fig 5.2.9-2

SCORING   *10 total points*

Scientific   *5 points*
○   Interobserver reliability
○   Intraobserver reliability
●   Universality
○●   Disease specificity

Clinical utility   *5 points*
●   Ease of application
●   Simplicity
●   Patient tolerability
●●   Affordability

●●●●●●●○○○   **7**

Reliability

Population tested in	Interobserver reliability	Intraobserver reliability
Not tested		

3   Lateral bending

Description
Movement in the coronal plane.

Interpretation
Normal range of motion: 15–20°

Clinical relevance
The overall tendency is that range of motion varies among individuals and decreases as age increases. Attention should be given to changes in serial exams or asymmetry.

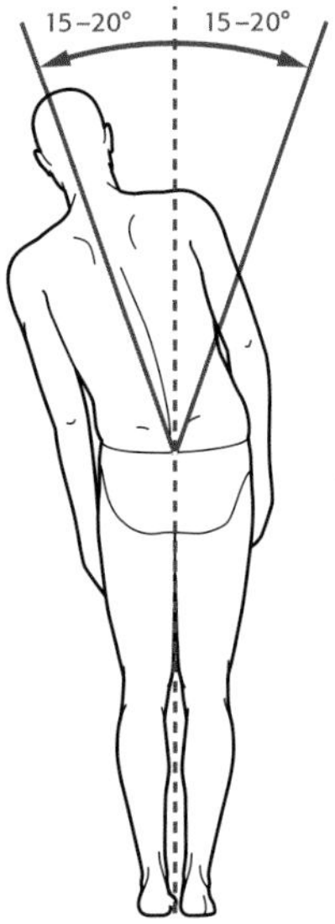

15–20°   15–20°

Fig 5.2.9-3

SCORING	10 total points

Scientific	5 points
○	Interobserver reliability
○	Intraobserver reliability
●	Universality
○●	Disease specificity

Clinical utility	5 points
●	Ease of application
●	Simplicity
●	Patient tolerability
●●	Affordability

●●●●●●●○○○   **7**

Reliability

Population tested in	Interobserver reliability	Intraobserver reliability
Not tested		

4   Rotation

Description
Movement in the axial plane.

Interpretation
Normal range of motion: 3–18°

Clinical relevance
The overall tendency is that range of motion varies among individuals and decreases as age increases. Attention should be given to changes in serial exams or asymmetry.

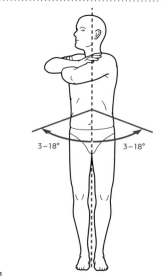

Fig 5.2.9-4

SCORING   *10 total points*

Scientific   *5 points*
○ Interobserver reliability
○ Intraobserver reliability
● Universality
○● Disease specificity

Clinical utility   *5 points*
● Ease of application
● Simplicity
● Patient tolerability
●● Affordability

●●●●●●●○○○   **7**

Reliability

Population tested in	Interobserver reliability	Intraobserver reliability
Not tested		

5.2.10   Spinal-pelvic sagittal balance

1   Pelvic incidence (PI)

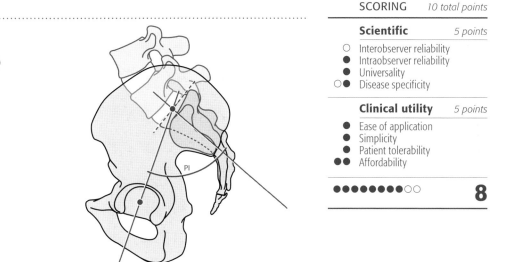

Description
The PI is defined as an angle created by a line drawn from the hip axis (HA) to the midpoint of the sacral end plate and a line perpendicular to the center of the sacral end plate. The HA is defined as the midpoint between the approximate centers of both femoral heads.

Interpretation
The greater the PI, the greater the lumbar lordosis that is necessary to maintain a neutral global sagittal alignment.

Clinical relevance
The measurement allows the clinician to determine the relative amount of lumbar lordosis that is needed to maintain balance.

SCORING   *10 total points*

Scientific   *5 points*
- ○ Interobserver reliability
- ● Intraobserver reliability
- ● Universality
- ○● Disease specificity

Clinical utility   *5 points*
- ● Ease of application
- ● Simplicity
- ● Patient tolerability
- ●● Affordability

●●●●●●●○○   **8**

Fig 5.2.10-1

Reliability

Population tested in	Interobserver reliability	Intraobserver reliability
Spinal and pelvic x-rays of asymptomatic patients (N = 160) measured twice 48 hours apart by ten experienced spine surgeons [1]	Manual -*	Manual +*

* The interobserver reliability and intraobserver reliability of these same measurements using a computer program is significantly higher.

References:
1. **Dimar JR 2nd, Carreon LY, Labelle H, et al** (2008) Intra- and inter-observer reliability of determining radiographic sagittal parameters of the spine and pelvis using a manual and a computer-assisted methods. *Eur Spine J;* 17:1373-1379.

2   Pelvic tilt (PT)

Description

PT is defined as the angle created by a vertical reference line through the hip axis (HA) and a line drawn from the midpoint of the sacral end plate to the HA.

Interpretation

PT has a (+) value when the midpoint of the sacrum is posterior to the vertical reference line and a (−) value when the midpoint of the sacrum is anterior to the vertical reference line.

Clinical relevance

The measurement allows the clinician to determine the relative amount of lumbar lordosis that is needed to maintain balance.

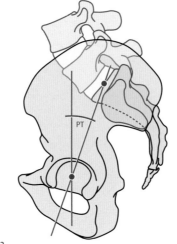

Fig 5.2.10-2

	SCORING	10 total points

Scientific	5 points
○ Interobserver reliability	
● Intraobserver reliability	
● Universality	
○● Disease specificity	

Clinical utility	5 points
● Ease of application	
● Simplicity	
● Patient tolerability	
●● Affordability	

●●●●●●●●○○   **8**

Reliability

Population tested in	Interobserver reliability	Intraobserver reliability
Spinal and pelvic x-rays of asymptomatic patients (N = 160) measured twice 48 hours apart by ten experienced spine surgeons [1]	Manual -*	Manual +*

* The interobserver reliability and intraobserver reliability of these same measurements using a computer program is significantly higher.

References:
1. **Dimar JR 2nd, Carreon LY, Labelle H, et al** (2008) Intra- and inter-observer reliability of determining radiographic sagittal parameters of the spine and pelvis using a manual and a computer-assisted methods. *Eur Spine J;* 17:1373-1379.

3   Sacral slope (SS)

Description
SS is defined as the angle created by a horizontal reference line and the sacral end plate.

Interpretation
The greater the slope, the greater the lumbar lordosis that is necessary to maintain neutral sagittal alignment.

Clinical relevance
The measurement allows the clinician to determine the relative amount of lumbar lordosis that is needed to maintain balance.

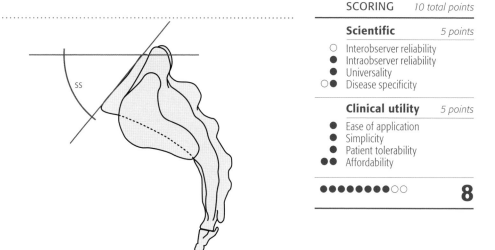

Fig 5.2.10-3

SCORING	10 total points
Scientific	5 points

- ○ Interobserver reliability
- ● Intraobserver reliability
- ● Universality
- ○● Disease specificity

Clinical utility	5 points

- ● Ease of application
- ● Simplicity
- ● Patient tolerability
- ●● Affordability

●●●●●●●●○○   **8**

Reliability

Population tested in	Interobserver reliability	Intraobserver reliability
Spinal and pelvic x-rays of asymptomatic patients (N = 160) measured twice 48 hours apart by ten experienced spine surgeons [1]	Manual -*	Manual +*

* The interobserver reliability and intraobserver reliability of these same measurements using a computer program is significantly higher.

References:
1. **Dimar JR 2nd, Carreon LY, Labelle H, et al** (2008) Intra- and inter-observer reliability of determining radiographic sagittal parameters of the spine and pelvis using a manual and a computer-assisted methods. *Eur Spine J;* 17:1373-1379.

4   Spinal canal stenosis

Description
The AP diameter in the x-ray of the
lumbar canals or the intraspinal canal
area measured in the MRI.

Interpretation
Severe: < 12 mm or intraspinal canal
area < 76 mm²

Moderate: < 100 mm²

Absolute measurements are not
valuable in all cases.

Clinical relevance
If clinically correlated, a small canal
diameter on a lateral x-ray may
indicate advanced stenosis.

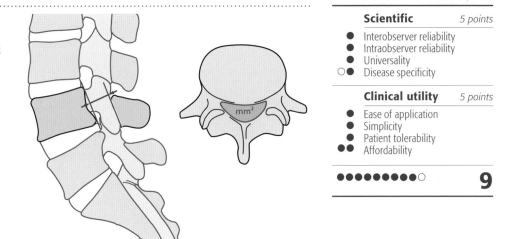

Fig 5.2.10-4

SCORING   *10 total points*

Scientific   *5 points*
● Interobserver reliability
● Intraobserver reliability
● Universality
○● Disease specificity

Clinical utility   *5 points*
● Ease of application
● Simplicity
● Patient tolerability
●● Affordability

●●●●●●●●●○   **9**

Reliability

Population tested in	Interobserver reliability	Intraobserver reliability
X-rays and axial CT of thoracolumbar burst fracture patients were evaluated twice by five observers [1]	Plain x-rays: -	Plain x-rays: -
	CT scans: +	CT scans: +

References:
1. Dai LY, Wang XY, Jiang LS (2008) Evaluation of traumatic spinal canal stenosis in thoracolumbar burst fractures. A comparison of three methods for measuring the percent canal occlusion. *Eur J Radiol;* 67:526-530.

5.2.11 Lumbar degenerative measurements

1 Disc height (normal values)

Description
Anterior disc height divided by the AP diameter of the cranial vertebral body multiplied by 100.

Interpretation
Normal values:
T12/L1: approximately 24%
L1/2: approximately 29%
L2/3: approximately 33%
L3/4: approximately 37%
L4/5: approximately 42%
L5/S1: approximately 41%

Clinical relevance
Radiographic disc heights loosely reflect the progression of degenerative disc disease and cervical spondylosis. While decreased disc height does correlate with the vertical diameter of the foramen, correlation with clinical presentation is necessary before treatment or additional imaging studies.

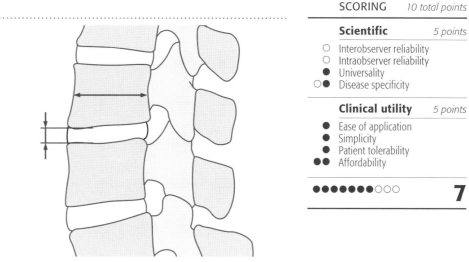

Fig 5.2.11-1

SCORING *10 total points*

Scientific *5 points*
○ Interobserver reliability
○ Intraobserver reliability
● Universality
○● Disease specificity

Clinical utility *5 points*
● Ease of application
● Simplicity
● Patient tolerability
●● Affordability

●●●●●●●○○○ **7**

Reliability

Population tested in	Interobserver reliability	Intraobserver reliability
Not tested		

2   Disc height

Description
The anterior and posterior edges of the adjacent vertebral bodies are defined as those points having the largest distance to the center of the vertebral body. Then, the distance of each of these four edges to the midplane of the disc is measured.

Interpretation
The sum of the two anterior distances is defined as actual anterior disc height, and the sum of the two posterior distances is defined as actual posterior disc height.

In vivo, this estimation becomes even more difficult due to the diurnal changes in disc. This actual height is compared to the respective height before degeneration.

Clinical relevance
Radiographic disc heights loosely reflect the progression of degenerative disc disease and cervical spondylosis. While decreased disc height does correlate with the vertical diameter of the foramen, correlation with clinical presentation is necessary before treatment or additional imaging studies.

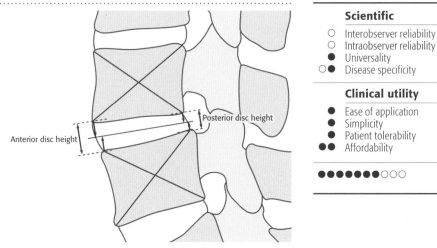

Fig 5.2.11-2

SCORING   *10 total points*

Scientific   *5 points*
○ Interobserver reliability
○ Intraobserver reliability
● Universality
○● Disease specificity

Clinical utility   *5 points*
● Ease of application
● Simplicity
● Patient tolerability
●● Affordability

●●●●●●●○○○   **7**

Reliability

Population tested in	Interobserver reliability	Intraobserver reliability
Not tested		

---

3 Osteophyte formation

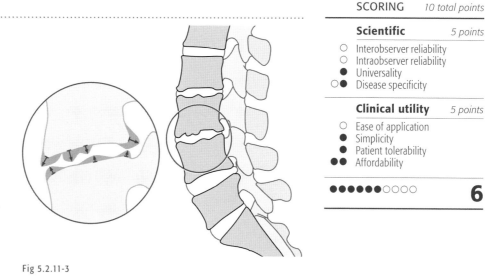

Fig 5.2.11-3

Description

The two anterior, two posterior, two right lateral, and two left lateral edges of the adjacent vertebral bodies are screened for osteophytes. Their number is counted and their length is measured along their long axis beginning at the former border of the vertebral body and ending at their tips.

The eight AP and lateral edges of the adjacent vertebral bodies are evaluated.

Interpretation

The sum of the heights of the four osteophytes.

Clinical relevance

Nonspecific osteophytosis generally indicates degenerative changes within the spinal column.

SCORING   *10 total points*

Scientific   *5 points*
- ○ Interobserver reliability
- ○ Intraobserver reliability
- ● Universality
- ○● Disease specificity

Clinical utility   *5 points*
- ○ Ease of application
- ● Simplicity
- ● Patient tolerability
- ●● Affordability

●●●●●●○○○○   **6**

Reliability

Population tested in	Interobserver reliability	Intraobserver reliability
Not tested		

4   Diffuse sclerosis

Description
It is assessed on the lateral x-rays only. The lower half of the upper vertebral body and the upper half of the lower vertebral body are each divided into regions.

Interpretation
The number of regions covered by sclerosis is counted.

Clinical relevance
Though often noted on radiographic review, this is generally a nonspecific finding and correlation with clinical presentation and other radiographic features are recommended.

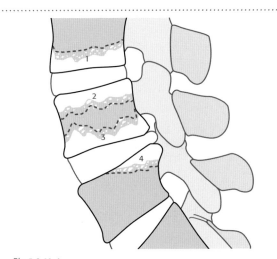

Fig 5.2.11-4

Reliability

Population tested in	Interobserver reliability	Intraobserver reliability
Not tested		

5.2.12 Congenital stenosis measurements

1   Facet angle

Description

The coronal reference plane marked by two points on the posterior wall of the vertebral body or intervertebral disc and two additional points are used to define the anteromedial and posterolateral margins of each facet joint. The facet joint angle is calculated relative to the coronal plane.

Interpretation

Upper limit of normal facet angulation: 45°

Normal range: 37.6–44.6°

More than 45° of both the left and right facet has a strong relationship with degenerative spondylolisthesis.

Clinical relevance

More sagittally aligned facets are thought to predispose the spinal segment to degenerative spondylolisthesis.

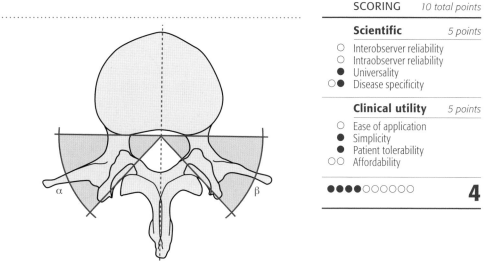

Fig 5.2.12-1

SCORING	10 total points

Scientific	5 points
○ Interobserver reliability	
○ Intraobserver reliability	
● Universality	
○● Disease specificity	

Clinical utility	5 points
○ Ease of application	
● Simplicity	
● Patient tolerability	
○○ Affordability	

●●●●○○○○○○   **4**

Reliability

Population tested in	Interobserver reliability	Intraobserver reliability
Not tested		

2   Facet tropism

Description
The difference between the angle of the right facet and the angle of the left facet at each level is measured.

Interpretation
No tropism: ≤6°

Mild: >6° and ≤10°

Moderate: >10° and ≤16°

Severe: >16°

Clinical relevance
An individual with facet joint angles at the level of the 4th and 5th lumbar vertebrae >45° relative to the coronal plane was 25 times more likely to have degenerative spondylolisthesis.

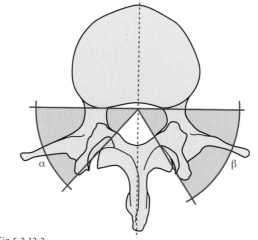

Fig 5.2.12-2

Reliability

Population tested in	Interobserver reliability	Intraobserver reliability
Not tested		

5.2.13 Vertebral body collapse in metastases of the thoracic and lumbar spine

1 Size of the lesion in the vertebrae

Description

The size and location of a metastatic tumor from T1 to L5 evaluated radiologically (CT scan).

Interpretation

The correlation between collapse and the following:
- Tumor size (in the vertebral body): x1
- Pedicule destruction: x2
- Posterior elements destruction: x3
- Costovertebral joint destruction: x4

Clinical relevance

The extent of osteolysis and destruction of the vertebral column and clinical symptoms correlates with a likelihood of further collapse and potentially neurological injury.

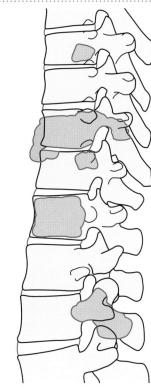

Fig 5.2.13-1

SCORING	10 total points
Scientific	5 points

○ Interobserver reliability
○ Intraobserver reliability
○ Universality
●● Disease specificity

Clinical utility	5 points

○ Ease of application
○ Simplicity
● Patient tolerability
○○ Affordability

●●●○○○○○○○ **3**

Reliability

Population tested in	Interobserver reliability	Intraobserver reliability
Not tested		

5.2.14   Infection measures—spine at risk in tuberculosis

1   Separation of the facet joints

Description
Measurement of the dislocation anterior superior of the facet joints compared to the adjacent superior and inferior segments on the apex of the curve in the sagittal x-ray view.

The facet joint dislocates at the level of the apex of the curve, causing instability and loss of alignment. In severe cases the separation can occur at two levels.

Interpretation
Comparison between the adjacent facet joints.

Clinical relevance
Substantial disparity of the facet appearance between affected and unaffected levels is suggestive of a destructive pathology and may warrant additional work-up.

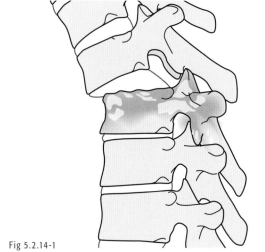

Fig 5.2.14-1

Reliability

Population tested in	Interobserver reliability	Intraobserver reliability
Not tested		

2   Posterior retropulsion of the diseased vertebral segments

Description
It is assessed by drawing two lines along the posterior surface of the normal vertebrae above and below the level of the lesion.

With progressive destruction, the remnants of the destroyed vertebral bodies were retropulsed.

Interpretation
Retropulsion is confirmed when bone at the involved level is seen posterior to the drawn lines.

Clinical relevance
Though this can be appreciated on standard x-rays, it is better visualized on advanced imaging with greater detail. This finding can suggest spinal instability and neurocompressive pathology.

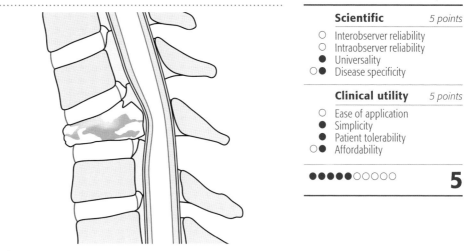

Fig 5.2.14-2

Reliability

Population tested in	Interobserver reliability	Intraobserver reliability
Not tested		

SCORING   *10 total points*

Scientific   *5 points*
○   Interobserver reliability
○   Intraobserver reliability
●   Universality
○● Disease specificity

Clinical utility   *5 points*
○   Ease of application
●   Simplicity
●   Patient tolerability
○● Affordability

●●●●●○○○○○   **5**

3   Lateral translation of the vertebral column

Description
A perpendicular line is drawn from the center of a pedicle of the first lower normal vertebra passing through the upper vertebra in AP x-rays.

Interpretation
Confirmed when this vertical line drawn through the middle of the pedicle of the first lower normal vertebra does not touch the pedicle of the first upper normal vertebra.

Clinical relevance
Suggests spinal instability warranting surgical stabilization.

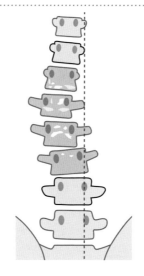

Fig 5.2.14-3

SCORING   *10 total points*

Scientific   *5 points*
○ Interobserver reliability
○ Intraobserver reliability
● Universality
○● Disease specificity

Clinical utility   *5 points*
● Ease of application
● Simplicity
● Patient tolerability
●● Affordability

●●●●●●●○○○   **7**

Reliability

Population tested in	Interobserver reliability	Intraobserver reliability
Not tested		

---

4   Toppling sign

Description
A line drawn along the anterior surface of the inferior vertebra will intersect the superior first normal vertebra above the middle of its anterior surface.

The separation of the facet joint allows the superior normal vertebral segment to tilt or topple, so that the anterior surface of the vertebra comes into contact with the superior surface of the vertebra below the level of the lesion.

Interpretation
Tilt or toppling occurs when the line intersects higher than the middle of the anterior surface of the first normal upper vertebra.

Clinical relevance
This finding indicates sagittal plane deformity with possible segmental instability.

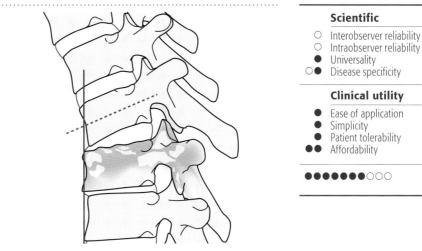

Fig 5.2.14-4

Reliability

Population tested in	Interobserver reliability	Intraobserver reliability
Not tested		

SCORING   *10 total points*

Scientific   *5 points*
○ Interobserver reliability
○ Intraobserver reliability
● Universality
○● Disease specificity

Clinical utility   *5 points*
● Ease of application
● Simplicity
● Patient tolerability
●● Affordability

●●●●●●●○○○   **7**

5.2.15   Deformity and kyphosis secondary to infection

1   Angle of coronal plane deformity

Description

Measured by drawing two lines, one on the superior surface of the uppermost involved vertebra and the other through the inferior surface of the lowermost involved vertebra, using the AP x-ray.

Interpretation

Measures only the angulations of the affected vertebrae.

Clinical relevance

This measurement indicates coronal plane deformity.

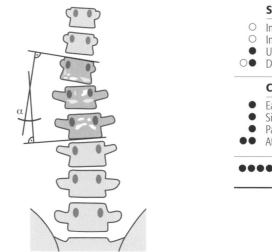

Fig 5.2.15-1

SCORING	10 total points
Scientific	5 points

- ○ Interobserver reliability
- ○ Intraobserver reliability
- ● Universality
- ○● Disease specificity

Clinical utility	5 points

- ● Ease of application
- ● Simplicity
- ● Patient tolerability
- ●● Affordability

●●●●●●●○○○   **7**

Reliability

Population tested in	Interobserver reliability	Intraobserver reliability
Not tested		

2 Angle of kyphosis

Description
Measured by drawing a line on the upper surface of the first normal vertebra above the lesion and another one through the lower surface of the first normal vertebra below the lesion.

Interpretation
Measures the localized segmental kyphosis.

Clinical relevance
This measurement indicates sagittal plane deformity.

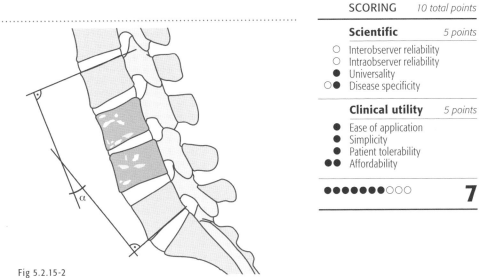

Fig 5.2.15-2

Reliability

Population tested in	Interobserver reliability	Intraobserver reliability
Not tested		

5.2.16   Osteoporosis measurements

5   Radiographic measurements
5.3   Deformity

5   Radiographic measurements

5.3   Deformity

Introduction

The ability to maintain neutral upright spinal alignment is intrinsic to the human condition because the species is in part defined by the ability to comfortably stand in an upright position for long periods of time. The human spine is a complex organ that has four major functions:

• Support the head, upper extremities, and torso
• Protect the spinal cord and nerve roots
• Control complex axial skeletal movements
• Transmit the body's weight to the hips by articulation with the pelvis

Neutral upright spinal alignment from the occiput to the pelvis in asymptomatic individuals is maintained in a relatively narrow range for maintenance of horizontal gaze, balance of the spine over the pelvis and femoral heads, and preservation of postural balance.

The spine is composed of regions with distinct alignment and biomechanical properties that contribute to global alignment. Although regional spinal curves vary widely from the occiput to the pelvis in asymptomatic individuals, global spinal alignment is maintained in a much narrower range for maintenance of horizontal gaze and balance of the spine over the pelvis and femoral heads. Spinal deformity is defined as a deviation from normal spinal alignment [1, 2]. Since the human condition is in part defined by the ability to comfortably stand upright and since the treatment of many patients with spinal disorders is directed at restoring this condition, spinal deformity needs to be defined in relation to neutral upright spinal alignment in asymptomatic individuals. Neutral upright spinal alignment in asymptomatic individuals is defined as standing with the knees and hips comfortably extended, the shoulders neutral or flexed, the neck neutral, and gaze horizontal. Analysis of spinal alignment involves both clinical and radiographic evaluation. Although there are a myriad of angles and displacements for measuring spinal alignment, the authors' analysis below offers a systematic approach to analyzing regional and global spinal alignment.

Clinical and radiographic evaluation of deformity

For the purpose of evaluating a spinal deformity:

- Clinical measurements are performed (facilitated with photographs) in a neutral upright position (standing with the knees and hips comfortably extended, the shoulders and neck neutral) and a forward bend position (standing with feet together, the knees comfortably extended, the hips and spine flexed, and the arms dependent with fingers and palms opposed).
- Occipitocervical and cervical angles and displacements are measured on standard standing anteroposterior and lateral cervical spine x-rays in a neutral upright position.
- Thoracic, lumbar, sacral, and pelvic angles and displacements, including spinal balance, are measured on standard standing anteroposterior and lateral long cassette x-rays in a neutral upright position (with the shoulders flexed for lateral x-rays).
- Side-bending (supine) and flexion/extension (standing) x-rays are obtained when appropriate for evaluating the flexibility of a deformity curve.

All upright imaging is performed barefoot. In patients with increased/decreased thoracic/lumbar vertebra, the anomalous vertebrae are included in the appropriate alignment-biomechanical zone. Leg length discrepancy less than 2 cm is ignored unless the leg length discrepancy significantly contributes to the spinal deformity. When the leg length discrepancy is greater than 2 cm, an appropriately thick lift is placed under the shorter leg.

Coronal spinal alignment	Neutral values Mean (1 SD) Adult > 18 years
Regional spinal alignment	
Occipitocervical junction angle: O–C2 apex	variable
Cervical angle: C2/3 disc–C6/7 disc apex	variable
Cervicothoracic junction angles: C7/T1 apex	variable
Proximal thoracic angle: T1/2 disc–T5 apex	< 20°
Main thoracic angle: T5/6 disc–T11/12 disc apex	< 20°
Thoracolumbar angle: T12/L1 apex	< 20°
Lumbar angle: L1/2 disc–L4/5 disc apex	< 20°
Lumbosacral junction angle: L5/S1 apex	variable
Shoulder tilt angle (ShTA)	1 (2 SD)
Angle of trunk inclination (ATI)	variable
Apical vertebral translation (AVT) (mm)	variable
Apical vertebral rotation (AVR)	< 5°–10°
Pelvic alignment	
Pelvic obliquity (PO)	< 8°
Leg length discrepancy (LLD) (mm)	6 (4 SD)
Global spinal alignment	
Interpupillary angle (IPA)	0 (1 SD)
Coronal spinal balance (mm)	
C7–S1 coronal vertical axis (CVA)	+4 (12 SD)
TT–S1 coronal vertical axis (CVA)	variable

Charles Kuntz IV (CKIV) neutral upright coronal spinal alignment guide: asymptomatic individuals

Table 5.3-1 Pooled estimates of the mean and variance of the neutral upright coronal spinal angles and displacements from the occiput to the pelvis. Assuming a normal distribution for coronal spinal angles and displacements in the population, the mean ± 1 SD includes approximately 68% of the population, the mean ± 2 SD includes approximately 95% of the population, and mean ± 2.5 SD includes approximately 98.5% of the population. Approximately 98.5% of asymptomatic individuals have coronal curves less than the estimated angle. For empty data cells there was little or no reproducible data [9] (with permission from the Mayfield Clinic).

Coronal alignment angles and displacements

By convention, coronal angles have a "+" value. Scoliotic curves are named for their convexity to the right or left. Coronal angulation of the head, shoulders, or pelvis is named for the elevated side: right is right up and left is left up.

Regional spinal alignment

Shoulder tilt angle (ShTA) is defined as the angle created by a horizontal reference line and a line drawn through the right and left coracoid processes. Trunk asymmetry (distortions of the torso) is measured using a scoliometer with the patient in a forward bend position (standing with feet together, the knees comfortably extended, the hips and spine flexed, and the arms dependent with fingers and palms opposed). The angle of trunk inclination (ATI) is the angle between a horizontal reference line and the plane across the back at the greatest elevation of a rib prominence or lumbar prominence. In contrast to radiographic measurements, the ShTA and ATI are clinical measurements of the effect of regional spinal deformity on trunk symmetry.

Occipitocervical (O–C2) curves are defined as having an apex from the occiput to C2. A coronal occipital reference line and the caudal end vertebrae are defined for measuring the Cobb angle [3].

Cervical coronal curves are defined as having an apex from the C2/3 disc to C6/7 disc and measured by the Cobb method from the end vertebrae [3].

The cervicothoracic junction angles are defined from C7 to T1. Cervicothoracic coronal curves are defined as having an apex from C7 to T1 and measured by the Cobb method from the end vertebrae [3].

Proximal thoracic (T1/2 disc to T5), main thoracic (T5/6 disc to T11/12 disc), thoracolumbar (T12 to L1), lumbar (L1/2 disc to L4/5 disc), and lumbosacral (L5 to S1) coronal curves are defined as having an apex in the above regions or zones and measured by the Cobb method from the end vertebrae [3]. The end vertebrae for all coronal curves are defined as the most cephalad and caudad vertebrae that maximally tilt into the concavity of the curve. The end vertebrae define the ends of the scoliotic curve. The cephalad end vertebra is the first vertebra in the cephalad direction from a curve apex whose superior surface is tilted maximally toward the concavity of the curve. The caudad end vertebra is the first vertebra in the caudad direction from a curve apex whose inferior surface is tilted maximally toward the concavity of the curve. The apical vertebra or disc of a curve is defined as the most horizontal and laterally deviated vertebra or disc of the curve [4]. Apical vertebral translation (AVT) is defined as the horizontal distance measured from the C7 plumb line to the center of the apical vertebral body or disc for proximal thoracic and main thoracic curves and from the central sacral vertical line (CSVL) to the center of the apical vertebral body or disc for thoracolumbar and lumbar curves [4]. The CSVL is defined as a vertical reference line drawn through the center of the S1 end plate. Apical vertebral rotation (AVR) is defined by the Nash-Moe classification system [4, 5]. Since AVR is defined on anteroposterior x-rays, AVR is included with the coronal alignment. Lateral olisthesis is defined by a modified Meyerding classification system [4, 6]. For lumbosacral coronal curves, the apical vertebra or disc is defined from L5 to S1. The cephalad end vertebra and a horizontal reference line are defined for measuring the Cobb angle (on supine side-bending x-rays the horizontal reference line may be reconstructed from the standing x-rays).

Pelvic alignment

Pelvic alignment and morphology are defined by the pelvic obliquity and leg length discrepancy. Pelvic obliquity (PO) is defined most frequently as the angle created by a horizontal reference line and a line drawn tangential to the top of the crests of the ilium or the base of the sulci of the S1 ala. Pelvic obliquity may result from an intrinsic sacropelvic deformity, leg length discrepancy, or a combination of both. Leg length discrepancy is defined as the vertical distance measured between horizontal lines drawn tangential to the top of the right and left femoral heads.

Global spinal alignment

Head tilt is defined by the interpupillary angle (IPA). The IPA is defined as the angle subtended by a horizontal reference line and the interpupillary line. The interpupillary line is defined by a line drawn though the center of the right and left pupils. In contrast to radiographic measurements, the IPA is a clinical measurement of total coronal deformity of the spine and the effect on horizontal gaze.

Coronal spinal balance is defined from the center of C7 and the midpoint of the thoracic trunk to the sacrum. The C7–S1 coronal vertical axis (C7–S1 CVA) is defined as the horizontal distance measured from a vertical plumb line centered in the middle of the C7 vertebral body to the CSVL. The C7–S1 CVA has a "+" value when the vertical plumb line is right of the CSVL and a "-" value when the vertical plumb line is left of the CSVL. The thoracic trunk–S1 coronal vertical axis (TT–S1 CVA) is defined as the horizontal distance measured from a vertical plumb line centered at the midpoint of the thorax to the CSVL (also known as thoracic trunk shift). The TT–S1 CVA is measured at the midpoint between the rib cage on the left and the rib cage on the right at the level of the main thoracic apical vertebra. If there is no main thoracic apical vertebra, the TT–S1 CVA is measured at the level of T9. The TT–S1 CVA has a "+" value when the vertical plumb line is right of the CVSL and a "-" value when the vertical plumb line is left of the CSVL.

Sagittal alignment angles and displacements

By convention, kyphosis has a "+" value and lordosis a "-" value.

Sagittal spinal alignment	Neutral values, Mean (1 SD), Adult > 18 years
Regional spinal alignment	
Occipitocervical junction angles	
O–C2	-14° (7°)
C1/2	-29° (7°)
Cervical lordosis: C2–7	-17° (14°)
Cervicothoracic junction angle: C6–T2	variable
Total thoracic kyphosis: T1–12	+45 (10)
Proximal thoracic kyphosis: T1–5	+14° (8°)
Main thoracic kyphosis: T4–12	+41° (11°)
Thoracolumbar junction angle: T10–L2	+6° (8°)
Total lumbosacral lordosis: T12/L1–S1	-62° (11°)
Lumbar lordosis: L1–5	-44° (11°)
Lumbosacral junction angles:	
L4–S1	variable
L4–5	-17° (5°)
L5/S1	-24° (6°)
Pelvic alignment	
Pelvic incidence (PI)	+54° (10°)
Pelvic tilt (PT)	+13° (6°)
Sacral slope (SS)	+41° (8°)
Global spinal alignment	
Chin-brow to vertical angle (CBVA)	-1° (3°)
Sagittal spinal balance	
C7–S1 sagittal vertical axis (SVA) (mm)	0° (24°)
T1–HA sagittal tilt angle (STA)	-1° (3°)
T9–HA STA	-11° (3°)

Charles Kuntz IV (CKIV) neutral upright sagittal spinal alignment guide: asymptomatic individuals

Table 5.3-2 Pooled estimates of the mean and variance of the neutral upright sagittal spinal angles and displacements from the occiput to the pelvis. Assuming a normal distribution for sagittal spinal angles and displacements in the population, the mean ± 1 SD includes approximately 68% of the population, the mean ± 2 SD includes approximately 95% of the population, and mean ± 2.5 SD includes approximately 98.5% of the population. For empty data cells there was little or no reproducible data [9] (with permission from the Mayfield Clinic).

Regional spinal alignment

Occipitocervical junction angles are defined from the occiput to C2. The O–C2 angle is defined as the angle subtended by the McGregor line and a line drawn parallel to the inferior end plate of C2. The McGregor line is drawn from the posterosuperior aspect of the hard palate to the most caudal point on the midline of the occipital curve [7]. The C1/2 angle is defined as the angle subtended by a line drawn parallel to the inferior aspect of C1 and a line drawn parallel to the inferior end plate of C2.

Cervical lordosis angles are defined from C2 to C7. The C2–7 angle is defined as the angle subtended by a line drawn parallel to the posterior border of the C2 vertebral body and a line drawn parallel to the posterior border of the C7 vertebral body.

Cervicothoracic junction angles are defined from C6 to T2, as measured by the Cobb method [3]. The C6–T2 angle is measured from the superior end plate of C6 to the inferior end plate of T2.

Thoracic kyphosis angles are defined from T1 to T12, as measured using the Cobb method [3]. Total thoracic kyphosis is measured from the superior end plate of T1 to the inferior end plate of T12. The proximal thoracic kyphosis is measured from the superior end plate of T1 to the inferior end plate of T5. The main thoracic kyphosis is measured from the superior end plate of T4 to the inferior end plate of T12.

Thoracolumbar junction angles are defined from T10 to L2, as measured using the Cobb method [3]. The T10–L2 angle is measured from the superior end plate of T10 to the inferior end plate of L2.

Lumbosacral lordosis angles are defined from T12/L1 to S1, as measured using the Cobb method [3]. Total lumbosacral lordosis is measured from either the inferior end plate of T12 or the superior end plate of L1 to the superior end plate of S1. Lumbar lordosis is measured from the superior end plate of L1 to the inferior end plate of L5.

Lumbosacral junction angles are measured from L4 to S1, as measured using the Cobb method [3]. The L4–S1 angle is measured from the superior end plate of L4 to the superior end plate of S1. The L4/5 angle is measured from the superior end plate of L4 to the superior end plate of L5. The L5/S1 angle is measured from the superior end plate of L5 to the superior end plate of S1.

Anterior and posterior olisthesis are defined by a modified Meyerding classification system [4, 6].

Pelvic alignment

Pelvic morphology and rotation are defined by the pelvic incidence (PI), pelvic tilt (PT), and sacral slope (SS). Pelvic incidence is a constant value unaffected by body posture. It is defined as an angle subtended by a line drawn from the hip axis to the midpoint of the sacral end plate and a line perpendicular to the center of the sacral end plate [8]. The hip axis (HA) is defined as the midpoint between the approximate centers of both femoral heads. As PI increases, lumbosacral lordosis must increase to maintain balanced sagittal global spinal alignment. In contrast to the PI, the SS and PT are posturally dependent values and change with rotation of the pelvis on the HA. SS is defined as the angle subtended by a horizontal reference line

and the sacral end plate. PT is defined as the angle subtended by a vertical reference line through the HA and a line drawn from the midpoint of the sacral end plate to the HA. PT has a "+" value when the midpoint of the sacrum is posterior to the vertical reference line and a "-" value when the midpoint of the sacrum is anterior to the vertical reference line. Geometrically, these pelvic angles produce the following equation: PI = SS + PT [8]. The pelvis rotates on the HA to help maintain balanced sagittal global spinal alignment.

Global spinal alignment

Chin-brow to vertical angle (CBVA) is defined as the angle subtended by a vertical reference line and a line drawn parallel to the chin and brow with the neck in neutral or fixed position and the knees and hips extended. In contrast to the radiographic measurements, the CBVA is a clinical measurement of the total sagittal deformity of the spine and the effect on horizontal gaze.

Sagittal spinal balance is defined from C7, T1, and T9 to the sacrum or HA. The C7–S1 sagittal vertical axis (C7–S1 SVA) is defined as the horizontal distance measured from a vertical plumb line centered in the middle of the C7 vertebral body to the posterior superior corner of the S1 end plate. The C7–S1 SVA has a "+" value when the vertical plumb line is anterior to the sacral reference point and a "-" value when the vertical plumb line is posterior to the sacral reference point. The T1–HA sagittal tilt angle (T1–HA STA) is defined as the angle subtended by a vertical reference line through the HA and a line drawn from the midpoint of the T1 vertebral body to the HA. The T9–HA STA is defined as the angle subtended by a vertical reference line through the HA and a line drawn from the midpoint of the T9 vertebral body to the HA. The T1–HA STA and T9–HA STA have a "+" value when the T1 or T9 midpoint is anterior to the HA vertical reference line and a "-" value when the T1 or T9 midpoint is posterior to the HA vertical reference line.

Summary

The spine needs to be evaluated in its entirety prior to formulating a treatment plan. The axial skeleton is composed of spinal regions or zones with distinct alignment and biomechanical properties that contribute to global spinal alignment. Although regional curves vary widely from the occiput to the pelvis in asymptomatic individuals, global spinal alignment is maintained in a much narrower range for maintenance of horizontal gaze and balance of the spine over the pelvis and femoral heads. Spinal deformity is defined as a deviation from normal spinal alignment. However, the practitioner should be mindful of numerous nonspinal factors that can severely affect spinal alignment. These can include limb length discrepancy, hip flexion contractures, and gluteal muscular atrophy, resulting in a fixed or dynamic deformity. The alignment of the body is dependent not only on the weight-bearing axis of the axial skeleton, but also the weight-bearing axis of the lower extremities. Pathology in either of these realms can adversely affect the other.

References

1. *Dorland's Illustrated Medical Dictionary.* (1994) 28th ed. W. B. Saunders: Philadelphia.
2. *Stedman's Medical Dictionary.* (2000) 27th ed. Lippincott Williams and Wilkins: Baltimore.
3. **Cobb JR** (1948) Outline for the study of scoliosis. *Edwards JW (ed), Instr Course Lect.* American Academy of Orthopaedic Surgeons, 261–275.
4. **O'Brien MF, Kuklo TR, Blanke KM, et al** (2004) *Radiographic Measurement Manual.* Memphis Tennessee: Medtronic Sofamor Danek, Inc.
5. **Nash CL, Jr., Moe JH** (1969) A study of vertebral rotation. *J Bone Joint Surg Am;* 51:223–229.
6. **Meyerding HW** (1931) Spondylolisthesis. *J Bone Joint Surg Am;* 13:39–48.
7. **McGregor M** (1948) The significance of certain measurements of the skull in the diagnosis of basilar impression. *Br J Radiol;* 21:171–181.
8. **Legaye J, Duval-Beaupere G, Hecquet J, et al** (1998) Pelvic incidence: a fundamental pelvic parameter for three-dimensional regulation of spinal sagittal curves. *Eur Spine J;* 7:99–103.
9. **Kuntz C, Levin LS, Ondra SL, et al** (2007) Neutral upright sagittal spinal alignment from the occiput to the pelvis in asymptomatic adults: a review and resynthesis of the literature. *J Neurosurg Spine;* 6:104–112.

5.3.1   Sagittal spinal alignment (cervical angles)

1   Cervical related angles

Description

a   Occipitocervical junction angle: The O–C2 angle is
defined as the angle subtended by the McGregor line
and a line drawn parallel to the inferior end plate of C2.
The McGregor line is drawn from the posterosuperior
aspect of the hard palate to the most caudal point on the
midline of the occipital curve.

b   Occipitocervical junction angle: The C1/2 angle is defined
as the angle subtended by a line drawn parallel to the
inferior aspect of C1 and a line drawn parallel to the
inferior end plate of C2.

c   Cervical lordosis: Cervical lordosis angles are defined
from C2 to C7. The C2–7 angle is defined as the angle
subtended by a line drawn parallel to the posterior
border of the C2 vertebral body and a line drawn
parallel to the posterior border of the C7 vertebral body.

d   Cervicothoracic junction angle: Cervicothoracic junction
angles are defined from C6 to T2, as measured by the
Cobb method. The C6–T2 angle is measured from the
superior end plate of C6 to the inferior end plate of T2.

Interpretation

The greater the angle, the greater the kyphosis or lordosis.

Clinical relevance

These measurements indicate the regional alignment
within the cervical spine and at the occipitocervical
junction.

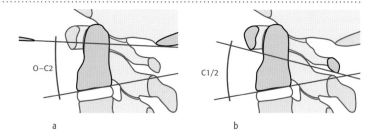

a   b

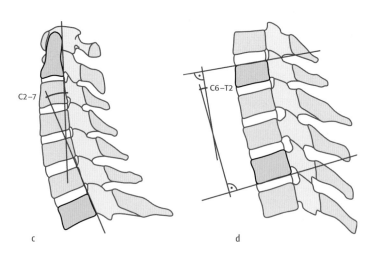

c   d

Fig 5.3.1-1a–d

a   SCORING   *10 total points*

Scientific   *5 points*

○ Interobserver reliability
○ Intraobserver reliability
● Universality
○● Disease specificity

Clinical utility   *5 points*

● Ease of application
● Simplicity
● Patient tolerability
●● Affordability

●●●●●●●○○○   **7**

b   SCORING   *10 total points*

Scientific   *5 points*

○ Interobserver reliability
○ Intraobserver reliability
● Universality
○● Disease specificity

Clinical utility   *5 points*

● Ease of application
● Simplicity
● Patient tolerability
●● Affordability

●●●●●●●○○○   **7**

c   SCORING   *10 total points*

Scientific   *5 points*

● Interobserver reliability
● Intraobserver reliability
● Universality
○● Disease specificity

Clinical utility   *5 points*

● Ease of application
● Simplicity
● Patient tolerability
●● Affordability

●●●●●●●●●○   **9**

d   SCORING   *10 total points*

Scientific   *5 points*

○ Interobserver reliability
○ Intraobserver reliability
● Universality
○● Disease specificity

Clinical utility   *5 points*

● Ease of application
● Simplicity
● Patient tolerability
●● Affordability

●●●●●●●○○○   **7**

Reliability

Population tested in	Interobserver reliability	Intraobserver reliability
Photographs of patients (N=36) with and without back pain (19 without) were visually assessed for cervical lordosis by 28 observers: chiropractors, physical therapists, physiatrists, rheumatologists, and orthopaedic surgeons [1]	-	-
X-rays of patients with cervical spondylotic myelopathy (N=20) were examined on three separate occasions for cervical lordosis using Cobb and posterior tangent methods by three independent observers: a spine fellowship-trained neurosurgeon, an orthopaedic surgeon in spine fellowship training, and a neurosurgical resident [2]	+	+

References:
1. Fedorak C, Ashworth N, Marshall J, et al (2003) Reliability of the visual assessment of cervical and lumbar lordosis: how good are we? *Spine (Phila Pa 1976);* 28:1857-1859.
2. Gwinn DE, Iannotti CA, Benzel EC, et al (2009) Effective lordosis: analysis of sagittal spinal canal alignment in cervical spondylotic myelopathy. *J Neurosurg Spine;* 11:667-672.

5.3.2   Sagittal spinal alignment (thoracic angles)

1   Thoracic related angles

Description

a   Total thoracic kyphosis: Thoracic kyphosis angles are defined from T1 to T12, as measured using the Cobb method. Total thoracic kyphosis is measured from the superior end plate of T1 to the inferior end plate of T12.

b   Proximal thoracic kyphosis: The proximal thoracic kyphosis is measured from the superior end plate of T1 to the inferior end plate of T5.

c   Main thoracic kyphosis: The main thoracic kyphosis is measured from the superior end plate of T4 to the inferior end plate of T12.

d   Thoracolumbar junction angle: Thoracolumbar junction angles are defined from T10 to L2, as measured using the Cobb method. The T10–L2 angle is measured from the superior end plate of T10 to the inferior end plate of L2.

Interpretation

The greater the Cobb angle, the greater the kyphosis or lordosis.

Clinical relevance

These measurements indicate the regional alignment within the thoracic spine and at the thoracolumbar junction.

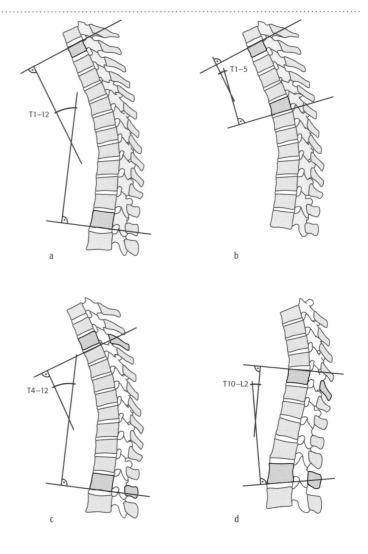

Fig 5.3.2-1a–d

a SCORING *10 total points*

Scientific *5 points*
- ● Interobserver reliability
- ● Intraobserver reliability
- ● Universality
- ○● Disease specificity

Clinical utility *5 points*
- ● Ease of application
- ● Simplicity
- ● Patient tolerability
- ●● Affordability

●●●●●●●●●○ **9**

b SCORING *10 total points*

Scientific *5 points*
- ○ Interobserver reliability
- ○ Intraobserver reliability
- ● Universality
- ○● Disease specificity

Clinical utility *5 points*
- ● Ease of application
- ● Simplicity
- ● Patient tolerability
- ●● Affordability

●●●●●●●○○○ **7**

c SCORING *10 total points*

Scientific *5 points*
- ● Interobserver reliability
- ● Intraobserver reliability
- ● Universality
- ○● Disease specificity

Clinical utility *5 points*
- ● Ease of application
- ● Simplicity
- ● Patient tolerability
- ●● Affordability

●●●●●●●●●○ **9**

d SCORING *10 total points*

Scientific *5 points*
- ○ Interobserver reliability
- ○ Intraobserver reliability
- ● Universality
- ○● Disease specificity

Clinical utility *5 points*
- ● Ease of application
- ● Simplicity
- ● Patient tolerability
- ●● Affordability

●●●●●●●○○○ **7**

Reliability

Population tested in	Interobserver reliability		Intraobserver reliability	
Preoperative and postoperative x-rays of adolescent idiopathic scoliosis patients (N = 30) were evaluated for various sagittal thoracic-related angles twice by three observers [1]	T2–5	-	T2–5	-
	T5–12	+	T5–12	+
	T2–12	+	T2–12	+
	T10 –L2	+	T10–L2	+
	T12–S1	+	T12–S1	+
Posteroanterior and lateral x-rays of adolescent idiopathic scoliosis patients (N = 10) were evaluated for various sagittal thoracic-related angles five times by two observers with differing levels of experience evaluating scoliosis [2]	Posteroanterior x-rays	+	Posteroanterior x-rays	+
	Lateral x-rays	-	Lateral x-rays	-

References:
1. Kuklo TR, Potter BK, O'Brien MF, et al (2005) Reliability analysis for digital adolescent idiopathic scoliosis measurements. *J Spinal Disord Tech;* 18:152-159.
2. Dang NR, Moreau MJ, Hill DL, et al (2005) Intra-observer reproducibility and interobserver reliability of the radiographic parameters in the Spinal Deformity Study Group's AIS Radiographic Measurement Manual. *Spine (Phila Pa 1976);* 30:1064-1069.

5.3.3   Sagittal spinal alignment (lumbar angles)

1   Lumbar related angles

Description
Lumbosacral lordosis angles are defined from T12/L1 to S1, as measured using the Cobb method.

a Total lumbosacral lordosis: Total lumbosacral lordosis is measured from either the inferior end plate of T12 or the superior end plate of L1 to the superior end plate of S1.

b Lumbar lordosis: Lumbar lordosis is measured from the superior end plate of L1 to the inferior end plate of L5.

Lumbosacral junction angles are measured from L4 to S1, as measured using the Cobb method [3].

c Lumbosacral junction angle: The L4–S1 angle is measured from the superior end plate of L4 to the superior end plate of S1.

d Lumbosacral junction angle The L4/5 angle is measured from the superior end plate of L4 to the superior end plate of L5.

e Lumbosacral junction angle: The L5/S1 angle is measured from the superior end plate of L5 to the superior end plate of S1.

Interpretation
The greater the Cobb angle, the greater the kyphosis or lordosis.

Clinical relevance
These measurements indicate the regional alignment within the lumbar spine and at the lumbosacral junction.

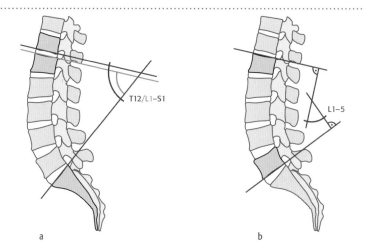

a   b

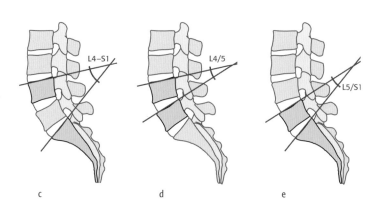

c   d   e

Fig 5.3.3-1a-e

a   SCORING   *10 total points*

Scientific   *5 points*

○ Interobserver reliability
○ Intraobserver reliability
● Universality
○● Disease specificity

Clinical utility   *5 points*

● Ease of application
● Simplicity
● Patient tolerability
●● Affordability

●●●●●●●○○○   **7**

b   SCORING   *10 total points*

Scientific   *5 points*

● Interobserver reliability
● Intraobserver reliability
● Universality
○● Disease specificity

Clinical utility   *5 points*

● Ease of application
● Simplicity
● Patient tolerability
●● Affordability

●●●●●●●●●○   **9**

c–e   SCORING   *10 total points*

Scientific   *5 points*

○ Interobserver reliability
○ Intraobserver reliability
● Universality
○● Disease specificity

Clinical utility   *5 points*

● Ease of application
● Simplicity
● Patient tolerability
●● Affordability

●●●●●●●○○○   **7**

Reliability

Population tested in	Interobserver reliability		Intraobserver reliability	
Photographs of patients (N=36) with and without back pain (19 without) were visually assessed for lumbar lordosis by 28 observers: chiropractors, physical therapists, physiatrists, rheumatologists, and orthopaedic surgeons [1]	-		-	
X-rays of patients with varying degrees of scoliosis (N=90) were assessed by different methods twice within two weeks for lumbar lordosis by three observers [2]	Cobb L1–5	+	Cobb L1–5	+
	Posterior tangent L1–5 method	+	Posterior tangent L1–5 method	+
	Cobb L1–S1 method	-	Cobb L1–S1 method	-
	Posterior tangent L1–S1 method	-	Posterior tangent L1–S1 method	-

References:
1. Fedorak C, Ashworth N, Marshall J, et al (2003) Reliability of the visual assessment of cervical and lumbar lordosis: how good are we? *Spine (Phila Pa 1976)*; 28:1857-1859.
2. Hong JY, Suh SW, Modi HN, et al (2010) Reliability analysis for radiographic measures of lumbar lordosis in adult scoliosis: a case-control study comparing 6 methods. *Eur Spine J*; 19:1551-1557.

5.3.4   Sagittal spinal alignment (pelvic alignment)

1   Pelvic incidence (PI)

Description

The PI is defined as an angle created by a line drawn from the hip axis (HA) to the midpoint of the sacral end plate and another line perpendicular to the center of the sacral end plate. The HA is defined as the midpoint between the approximate centers of both femoral heads.

Interpretation

The greater the PI, the greater the lumbar lordosis that is necessary to maintain a neutral global sagittal alignment.

Clinical relevance

The measurement allows the clinician to determine the relative amount of lumbar lordosis that is needed to maintain global sagittal spinal balance.

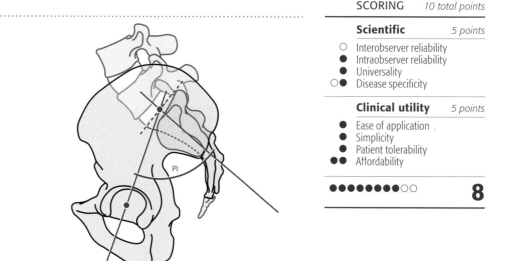

Fig 5.3.4-1

SCORING   *10 total points*

Scientific	*5 points*
○	Interobserver reliability
●	Intraobserver reliability
○●	Universality
○●	Disease specificity

Clinical utility	*5 points*
●	Ease of application
●	Simplicity
●	Patient tolerability
●●	Affordability

●●●●●●●●○○   **8**

Reliability

Population tested in	Interobserver reliability	Intraobserver reliability
Spinal and pelvic x-rays of asymptomatic patients (N = 160) measured twice 48 hours apart by ten experienced spine surgeons [1]	Manual -*	Manual +*

* The interobserver reliability and intraobserver reliability of these same measurements using a computer program is significantly higher.

References:
1. **Dimar JR 2nd, Carreon LY, Labelle H, et al** (2008) Intra- and inter-observer reliability of determining radiographic sagittal parameters of the spine and pelvis using a manual and a computer-assisted methods. *Eur Spine J;* 17:1373-1379.

2   Pelvic tilt (PT)

Description

PT is defined as the angle created by a vertical reference line through the hip axis (HA) and a line drawn from the midpoint of the sacral end plate to the HA.

Interpretation

PT has a "+" value when the midpoint of the sacrum is posterior to the vertical reference line and a (−) value when the midpoint of the sacrum is anterior to the vertical reference line.

Clinical relevance

The measurement allows the clinician to determine the relative rotation of the pelvis on the HA.

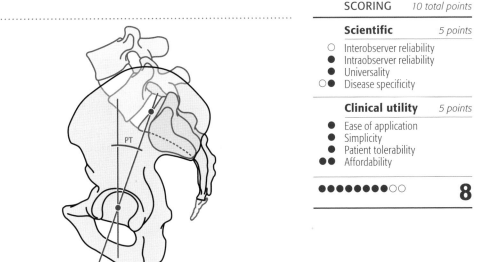

Fig 5.3.4-2

SCORING	10 total points

Scientific   5 points

○ Interobserver reliability
● Intraobserver reliability
● Universality
○● Disease specificity

Clinical utility   5 points

● Ease of application
● Simplicity
● Patient tolerability
●● Affordability

●●●●●●●●○○   **8**

Reliability

Population tested in	Interobserver reliability	Intraobserver reliability
Spinal and pelvic x-rays of asymptomatic patients (N = 160) measured twice 48 hours apart by ten experienced spine surgeons [1]	Manual -*	Manual +*

* The interobserver reliability and intraobserver reliability of these same measurements using a computer program is significantly higher.

References:
1. **Dimar JR 2nd, Carreon LY, Labelle H, et al** (2008) Intra- and inter-observer reliability of determining radiographic sagittal parameters of the spine and pelvis using a manual and a computer-assisted methods. *Eur Spine J;* 17:1373-1379.

3   Sacral slope (SS)

Description
SS is defined as the angle created by a horizontal reference line and the sacral end plate.

Interpretation
The greater the slope, the greater the lumbar lordosis that is necessary to maintain neutral global sagittal alignment.

Clinical relevance
The measurement is influenced by the pelvic incidence and pelvic tilt. It allows the clinician to determine the relative amount of lumbar lordosis that is needed to maintain global sagittal spinal balance.

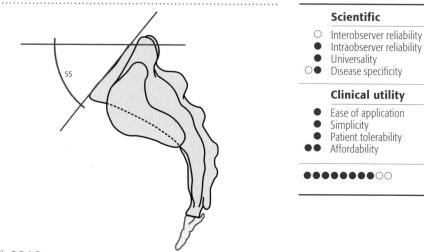

Fig 5.3.4-3

Reliability

Population tested in	Interobserver reliability	Intraobserver reliability
Spinal and pelvic x-rays of asymptomatic patients (N = 160) measured twice 48 hours apart by ten experienced spine surgeons [1]	Manual -*	Manual +*

* The interobserver reliability and intraobserver reliability of these same measurements using a computer program is significantly higher.

References:
1. Dimar JR 2nd, Carreon LY, Labelle H, et al (2008) Intra- and inter-observer reliability of determining radiographic sagittal parameters of the spine and pelvis using a manual and a computer-assisted methods. *Eur Spine J;* 17:1373-1379.

5.3.5   Sagittal spinal alignment (global spinal alignment)

1   Chin-brow to vertical angle (CBVA)

Description
CBVA is defined as the angle created by a vertical reference line and a line drawn parallel to the chin and brow with the neck in neutral or fixed position and the knees and hips extended. This is determined by clinical assessment of the patient, not by an x-ray.

Interpretation
The greater the angle, the more kyphotic or more positive the sagittal balance.

Clinical relevance
This measurement is a clinical indicator of global sagittal spinal alignment.

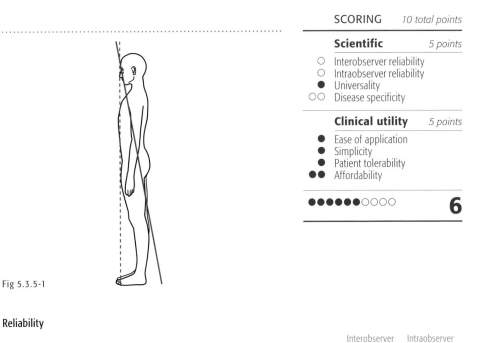

Fig 5.3.5-1

SCORING   *10 total points*

Scientific   *5 points*
○   Interobserver reliability
○   Intraobserver reliability
●   Universality
○○ Disease specificity

Clinical utility   *5 points*
●   Ease of application
●   Simplicity
●   Patient tolerability
●● Affordability

●●●●●●○○○○   **6**

Reliability

Population tested in	Interobserver reliability	Intraobserver reliability
Not tested		

2   Sagittal spinal balance: C7–S1 sagittal vertical axis (SVA) (mm)

Description

The C7–S1 sagittal vertical axis (C7–S1 SVA) is defined as the horizontal distance measured from a vertical plumb line centered in the middle of the C7 vertebral body to the posterior superior corner of the S1 end plate.

Interpretation

When the plumb line is anterior to the posterior superior corner of the S1 end plate, this is deemed positive sagittal balance. When it is posterior to the posterior superior corner of the S1 end plate, this is deemed negative sagittal balance. This is quantified by the actual distance from the plumb line to the posterior superior corner of the S1 end plate.

Clinical relevance

This measurement is an indicator of global sagittal spinal balance.

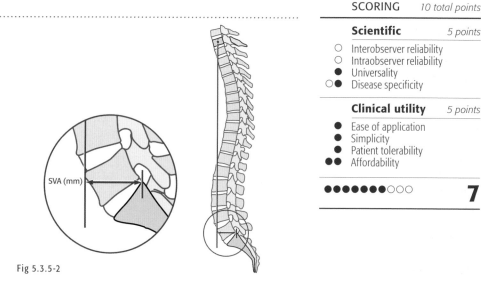

Fig 5.3.5-2

Reliability

Population tested in	Interobserver reliability	Intraobserver reliability
X-rays of neuromuscular scoliosis patients (N=48) were evaluated for C7 balance twice by seven observers: two attending spine surgeons, two attending pediatric orthopedists, one pediatrician experienced in spinal cord injury, one spine fellow, and one resident [1]	-	-

References:
1. Gupta MC, Wijesekera S, Sossan A, et al (2007) Reliability of radiographic parameters in neuromuscular scoliosis. *Spine;* 32:691-695.

---

3   Sagittal spinal balance: T1–HA sagittal tilt angle (STA)

Description

The T1–HA sagittal tilt angle (T1–HA STA) is defined as the angle created by a vertical reference line through the hip axis (HA) and another line drawn from the midpoint of the T1 vertebral body to the HA.

Interpretation

When the T1 midpoint is anterior to the HA, this indicates a positive measurement. When the T1 midpoint is posterior to the HA, this indicates a negative measurement.

Clinical relevance

This measurement is an indicator of global sagittal spinal balance.

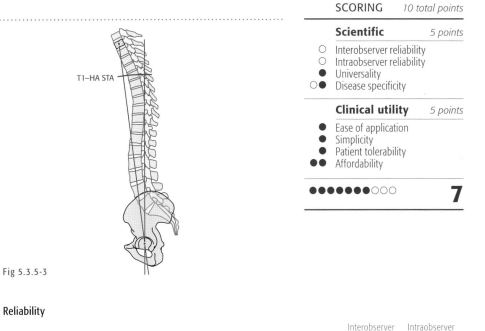

T1–HA STA

Fig 5.3.5-3

Reliability

Population tested in	Interobserver reliability	Intraobserver reliability
Not tested		

4   Sagittal spinal balance: T9–HA sagittal tilt angle (STA)

Description
The T9–HA sagittal tilt angle
(T9–HA STA) is defined as the angle
created by a vertical reference line
through the hip axis (HA) and
a line drawn from the midpoint of
the T9 vertebral body to the HA.

Interpretation
When the T9 midpoint is anterior to
the HA, this indicates a positive
measurement. When the T9 midpoint
is posterior to the HA, this indicates a
negative measurement.

Clinical relevance
This measurement is an indicator of
global sagittal spinal balance.

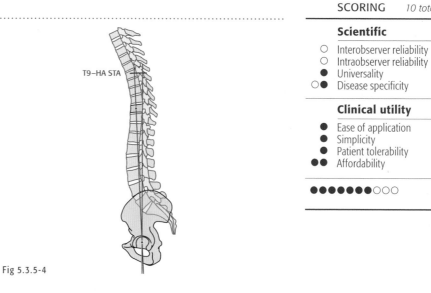

T9–HA STA

Fig 5.3.5-4

SCORING   *10 total points*

Scientific	*5 points*
○	Interobserver reliability
○	Intraobserver reliability
●	Universality
○●	Disease specificity

Clinical utility	*5 points*
●	Ease of application
●	Simplicity
●	Patient tolerability
●●	Affordability

●●●●●●●○○○   **7**

Reliability

Population tested in	Interobserver reliability	Intraobserver reliability
Not tested		

5   Seattle angle [1]

Description
When planning an osteotomy to restore sagittal balance of the spine, the Seattle angle is between the femoral axis and the line from C7 to the proposed osteotomy site. This requires a full spine lateral x-ray that includes the superior portion of the femoral axis.

Interpretation
The greater the Seattle angle, the greater the amount of lordosis restoration that is required. By utilizing the femoral axis, this angle accounts for hip flexion contractures which may contribute to sagittal imbalance.

Clinical Relevance
This angle reflects the severity of global sagittal imbalance by also accounting for the effect of hip flexion contracture.

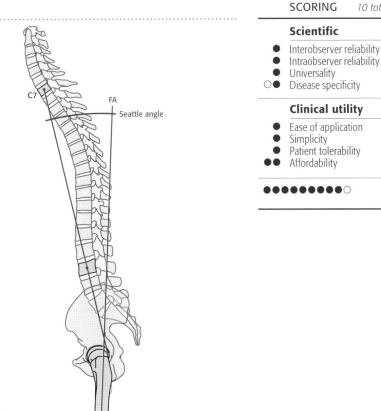

Fig 5.3.5-5

	SCORING	10 total points
	Scientific	5 points
●	Interobserver reliability	
●	Intraobserver reliability	
●	Universality	
○●	Disease specificity	
	Clinical utility	5 points
●	Ease of application	
●	Simplicity	
●	Patient tolerability	
●●	Affordability	

●●●●●●●●●○   **9**

Reliability

Population tested in	Interobserver reliability	Intraobserver reliability
Patients (N = 30) who required spinal osteotomies to regain sagittal balance were measured twice 6 weeks apart by a spine surgeon and musculoskeletal radiologist [1]	+	+

References:
1. Elgafy H, Bransford R, Semaan H, et al (2011) Clinical and radiographic evaluation of sagittal imbalance: a new radiographic assessment. *Am J Orthop;* 40:E30-34.

5.3.6   Coronal spinal alignment (cervical angles)

---

1   Cervical related angles

....

Description

a Occipitocervical junction angle: O–C2 apex Occipitocervical
(O–C2) curves are defined as having an apex from the
occiput to C2. A coronal occipital reference line and the
caudal end vertebrae are defined for measuring the Cobb
angle.

b Cervical angle: C2/3 disc–C6/7 disc apex Cervical coronal
curves are defined as having an apex from the C2/3 disc
to C6/7 disc and measured by the Cobb method from the
end vertebrae.

c Cervicothoracic junction angle: C7/T1 apex Cervicothoracic
coronal curves are defined as having an apex from C7 to
T1 and measured by the Cobb method from the end
vertebrae.

Interpretation
The greater the Cobb angle, the greater the scoliosis.

Clinical relevance
These measurements indicate the regional alignment
within the cervical spine and occipitocervical junction.

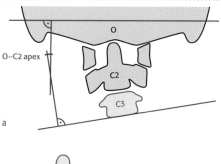

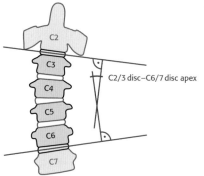

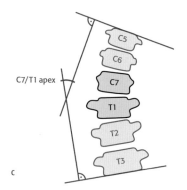

Fig 5.3.6-1a–c

a   SCORING   *10 total points*

Scientific   *5 points*

○ Interobserver reliability
○ Intraobserver reliability
● Universality
○● Disease specificity

Clinical utility   *5 points*

● Ease of application
● Simplicity
● Patient tolerability
●● Affordability

●●●●●●●○○○   **7**

b   SCORING   *10 total points*

Scientific   *5 points*

○ Interobserver reliability
○ Intraobserver reliability
● Universality
○● Disease specificity

Clinical utility   *5 points*

● Ease of application
● Simplicity
● Patient tolerability
●● Affordability

●●●●●●●○○○   **7**

c   SCORING   *10 total points*

Scientific   *5 points*

○ Interobserver reliability
○ Intraobserver reliability
● Universality
○● Disease specificity

Clinical utility   *5 points*

● Ease of application
● Simplicity
● Patient tolerability
●● Affordability

●●●●●●●○○○   **7**

Reliability

Population tested in	Interobserver reliability	Intraobserver reliability
Not tested		

5.3.7   Coronal spinal alignment (thoracic angles)

1   Thoracic related angles

Description

Thoracic coronal angles are defined from T1 to T12, as measured using the Cobb method from the end vertebrae.

a   **Proximal thoracic angle: T1–5 apex** proximal thoracic curves.

b   **Main thoracic angle: T5–12 apex** main thoracic curves.

c   **Thoracolumbar angle: T10–L2 apex** thoracolumbar curves.

Interpretation

The greater the Cobb angle, the greater the scoliosis.

Clinical relevance

These measurements indicate the magnitude of coronal deformity.

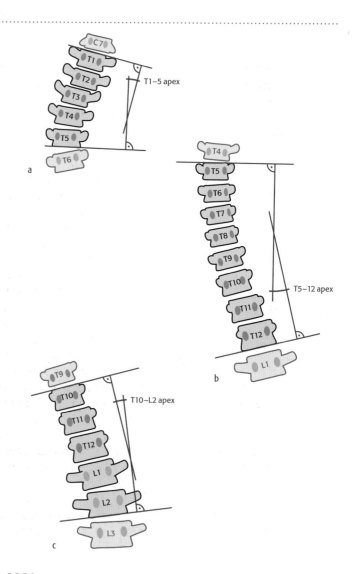

Fig 5.3.7-1a–c

a SCORING *10 total points*

Scientific *5 points*

○ Interobserver reliability
○ Intraobserver reliability
● Universality
○● Disease specificity

Clinical utility *5 points*

● Ease of application
● Simplicity
● Patient tolerability
●● Affordability

●●●●●●●○○○ **7**

b SCORING *10 total points*

Scientific *5 points*

● Interobserver reliability
● Intraobserver reliability
● Universality
○● Disease specificity

Clinical utility *5 points*

● Ease of application
● Simplicity
● Patient tolerability
●● Affordability

●●●●●●●●●○ **9**

c SCORING *10 total points*

Scientific *5 points*

○ Interobserver reliability
○ Intraobserver reliability
● Universality
○● Disease specificity

Clinical utility *5 points*

● Ease of application
● Simplicity
● Patient tolerability
●● Affordability

●●●●●●●○○○ **7**

Reliability

Population tested in	Interobserver reliability		Intraobserver reliability	
Preoperative and postoperative x-rays of adolescent idiopathic scoliosis patients (N = 30) were evaluated for various coronal thoracic-related angles twice by three observers [1]	Main thoracic	+	Main thoracic	+

References:
1. Kuklo TR, Potter BK, O'Brien MF, et al (2005) Reliability analysis for digital adolescent idiopathic scoliosis measurements. *J Spinal Disord Tech;* 18:152-159.

5.3.8   Coronal spinal alignment (lumbar angles)

1   Lumbar related angles

Description
Lumbar angles are defined by measuring the angles of the proximal and distal end plates of the curve, using the Cobb method from the end vertebrae.

a Lumbar angle: L1/2 disc–L4/5 disc apex

b Lumbosacral junction angle: L5/S1 apex

Interpretation
The greater the Cobb angle, the greater the scoliosis.

Clinical relevance
These measurements indicate the magnitude of coronal deformity.

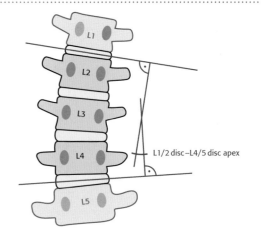

a

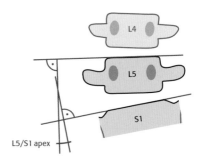

b

Fig 5.3.8-1a–b

a   SCORING   *10 total points*

Scientific   *5 points*

- ○ Interobserver reliability
- ○ Intraobserver reliability
- ● Universality
- ○● Disease specificity

Clinical utility   *5 points*

- ● Ease of application
- ● Simplicity
- ● Patient tolerability
- ●● Affordability

●●●●●●●○○○   **7**

b   SCORING   *10 total points*

Scientific   *5 points*

- ○ Interobserver reliability
- ○ Intraobserver reliability
- ● Universality
- ○● Disease specificity

Clinical utility   *5 points*

- ● Ease of application
- ● Simplicity
- ● Patient tolerability
- ●● Affordability

●●●●●●●○○○   **7**

Reliability

Population tested in	Interobserver reliability	Intraobserver reliability
Not tested		

5.3.9   Coronal spinal alignment (lumbosacral related angles)

1   Apical vertebral translation (AVT)

Description

Apical vertebral translation (AVT) is defined as the horizontal distance measured from the C7 plumb line to the center of the apical vertebral body or disc for proximal thoracic and main thoracic curves, and from the central sacral vertical line (CSVL) to the center of the apical vertebral body or disc for thoracolumbar and lumbar curves.

Interpretation

The greater the distance, the greater the coronal shift.

Clinical relevance

This measurement indicates the severity of the translational component of the deformity.

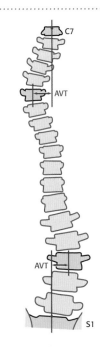

Fig 5.3.9-1

SCORING   *10 total points*

Scientific   *5 points*
- ● Interobserver reliability
- ● Intraobserver reliability
- ● Universality
- ○● Disease specificity

Clinical utility   *5 points*
- ● Ease of application
- ● Simplicity
- ● Patient tolerability
- ●● Affordability

●●●●●●●●●○   **9**

Reliability

Population tested in	Interobserver reliability	Intraobserver reliability
Preoperative and postoperative x-rays of adolescent idiopathic scoliosis patients (N = 30) were evaluated for apical vertebral translation twice by three observers [1]	+	+
Posteroanterior and lateral x-rays of adolescent idiopathic scoliosis patients (N = 10) were evaluated for apical vertebral translation five times by two observers with differing levels of experience evaluating scoliosis [2]	Posteroanterior x-rays + Lateral x-rays -	Posteroanterior x-rays + Lateral x-rays -

References:
1. Kuklo TR, Potter BK, O'Brien MF, et al (2005) Reliability analysis for digital adolescent idiopathic scoliosis measurements. *J Spinal Disord Tech;* 18:152-159.
2. Dang NR, Moreau MJ, Hill DL, et al (2005) Intra-observer reproducibility and interobserver reliability of the radiographic parameters in the Spinal Deformity Study Group's AIS Radiographic Measurement Manual. *Spine (Phila Pa 1976);* 30:1064-1069.

2   Apical vertebral rotation (AVR)

Description

Traditionally, this had been measured by trigonometric conversion of vertebral landmarks on an anterior posterior x-ray. However, it is now most easily measured on advanced imaging axial views by measuring the AP axis of the patient's body against the AP axis of the vertebral body.

Interpretation

The greater the angle, the greater the rotation.

Clinical relevance

This measurement indicates the severity of the rotational component of the deformity.

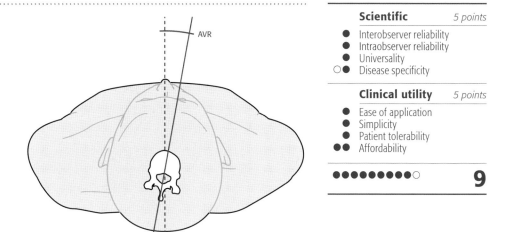

Fig 5.3.9-2

SCORING	10 total points
Scientific	5 points

- ● Interobserver reliability
- ● Intraobserver reliability
- ● Universality
- ○● Disease specificity

Clinical utility	5 points

- ● Ease of application
- ● Simplicity
- ● Patient tolerability
- ●● Affordability

●●●●●●●●●○   **9**

Reliability

Population tested in	Interobserver reliability	Intraobserver reliability
Posteroanterior and lateral x-rays of adolescent idiopathic scoliosis patients (N = 10) were evaluated for apical vertebral rotation five times by two observers with differing levels of experience evaluating scoliosis [1]	Posteroanterior x-rays + Lateral x-rays -	Posteroanterior x-rays + Lateral x-rays -
Preoperative CT scans of non-congenital scoliosis patients (N = 25) were measured by a CT scan method and by Ho's method [2]	+	+

References:
1. Dang NR, Moreau MJ, Hill DL, et al (2005) Intra-observer reproducibility and interobserver reliability of the radiographic parameters in the Spinal Deformity Study Group's AIS Radiographic Measurement Manual. *Spine (Phila Pa 1976);* 30:1064-1069.
2. Doi T, Kido S, Kuwashima U, et al (2011) A new method for measuring torsional deformity in scoliosis. *Scoliosis;* 6:7.

5.3.10   Coronal spinal alignment (pelvic alignment)

1   Pelvic obliquity (PO)

Description
Pelvic obliquity (PO) is defined most frequently as the angle created by a horizontal reference line and a line drawn tangential to the top of the crests of the ilium or the base of the sulci of the S1 alae.

Interpretation
The greater the angle, the greater the pelvic obliquity.

Clinical relevance
This measurement is one indicator of the magnitude of pelvic asymmetry.

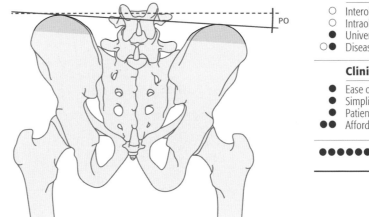

Fig 5.3.10-1

SCORING   *10 total points*

Scientific   *5 points*
- ○ Interobserver reliability
- ○ Intraobserver reliability
- ● Universality
- ○● Disease specificity

Clinical utility   *5 points*
- ● Ease of application
- ● Simplicity
- ● Patient tolerability
- ●● Affordability

●●●●●●●○○○   **7**

Reliability

Population tested in	Interobserver reliability	Intraobserver reliability
X-rays of patients to be treated for pelvic obliquity (N =36) were assessed by line of eburnation and the intersulcate line by four blinded raters [1]	Intersulcate line + Line of eburnation -	Intersulcate line + Line of eburnation -
X-rays of neuromuscular scoliosis patients (N = 48) were evaluated for C7 balance twice by seven observers: two attending spine surgeons, two attending pediatric orthopedists, one pediatrician experienced in spinal cord injury, one spine fellow, and one resident [2]	-	-

References:
1. Fann AV, Lee R, Verbois GM (1999) The reliability of postural x-rays in measuring pelvic obliquity. *Arch Phys Med Rehabil;* 80:458-461.
2. Gupta MC, Wijesekera S, Sossan A, et al (2007) Reliability of radiographic parameters in neuromuscular scoliosis. *Spine;* 32:691-695.

2 Leg length discrepancy (LLD)

Description
Leg length discrepancy (LLD) is defined as the vertical distance measured between horizontal lines drawn tangential to the top of the right and left femoral heads.

Interpretation
The difference in vertical height between these lines represents the leg length discrepancy.

Clinical relevance
Leg length discrepancy has multiple etiologies and if severe enough, can affect pelvic and spinal alignment.

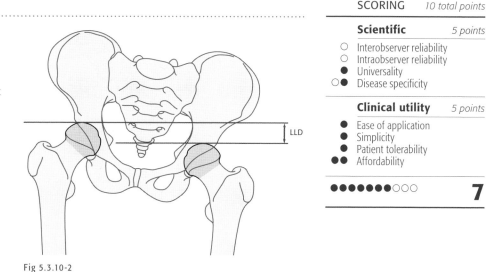

Fig 5.3.10-2

SCORING   *10 total points*

Scientific   *5 points*
○ Interobserver reliability
○ Intraobserver reliability
● Universality
○● Disease specificity

Clinical utility   *5 points*
● Ease of application
● Simplicity
● Patient tolerability
●● Affordability

●●●●●●●○○○   **7**

Reliability

Population tested in	Interobserver reliability	Intraobserver reliability
Not tested		

5.3.11   Coronal spinal alignment (global spinal alignment)

---

1   Head tilt angle: interpupillary angle (IPA)

....

Description
The IPA is defined as the angle created by a horizontal reference line and the interpupillary line based on clinical evaluation.

Interpretation
The greater the angle, the larger the coronal deformity.

Clinical relevance
This measurement is a clinical indicator of global coronal spinal alignment.

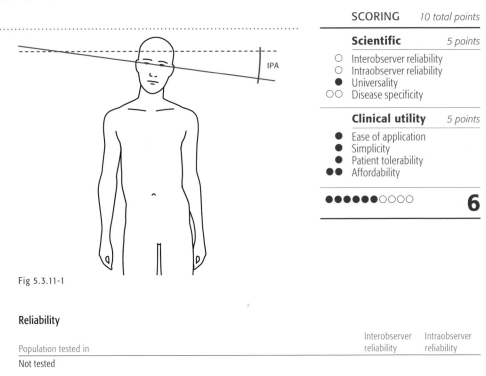

Fig 5.3.11-1

SCORING	10 total points
Scientific	5 points

○ Interobserver reliability
○ Intraobserver reliability
● Universality
○○ Disease specificity

Clinical utility	5 points

● Ease of application
● Simplicity
● Patient tolerability
●● Affordability

●●●●●●○○○○   **6**

Reliability

Population tested in	Interobserver reliability	Intraobserver reliability
Not tested		

2   Shoulder tilt angle

Description
The shoulder tilt angle is the angle created by a horizontal reference line and the intershoulder line based on clinical evaluation.

Interpretation
The greater the angle, the larger the coronal deformity.

Clinical relevance
This measurement is a clinical indicator of regional spinal alignment.

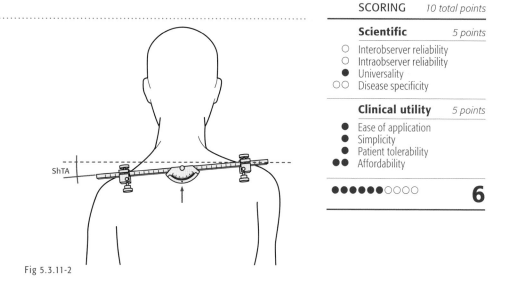

ShTA

Fig 5.3.11-2

SCORING   *10 total points*

Scientific   *5 points*
○ Interobserver reliability
○ Intraobserver reliability
● Universality
○○ Disease specificity

Clinical utility   *5 points*
● Ease of application
● Simplicity
● Patient tolerability
●● Affordability

●●●●●●○○○○   **6**

Reliability

Population tested in	Interobserver reliability	Intraobserver reliability
Not tested		

3   Coronal spinal balance: C7–S1 coronal vertical axis (CVA) (mm)

Description
The C7–S1 coronal vertical axis (C7–S1 CVA) is defined as the horizontal distance measured from a vertical plumb line centered in the middle of the C7 vertebral body to the central sacral vertical line (CSVL).

Interpretation
The C7–S1 CVA has a "+" value when the vertical plumb line is right of the CSVL and a (−) value when the vertical plumb line is left of the CSVL.

Clinical relevance
This measurement is an indicator of global coronal spinal balance.

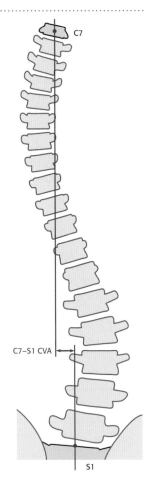

Fig 5.3.11-3

SCORING	10 total points

Scientific	5 points
○ Interobserver reliability	
○ Intraobserver reliability	
● Universality	
○● Disease specificity	

Clinical utility	5 points
● Ease of application	
● Simplicity	
● Patient tolerability	
●● Affordability	

●●●●●●●○○○   **7**

Reliability

Population tested in	Interobserver reliability	Intraobserver reliability
Not tested		

4   Thoracic trunk shift

Description
This is measured on an AP or PA scoliosis x-ray. A horizontal line is drawn through the apical thoracic vertebra. Along this horizontal line, the midpoint is identified between the lateral margins of the right and left rib cage. From this midpoint, the perpendicular vertical line is drawn. This line is known as the vertebral trunk reference line (VTRL). The distance between this line and the center sacral vertebral line is the thoracic trunk shift.

Interpretation
The greater the value, the greater the coronal shift of the thoracic spine. If the shift is to the patient's right, the value will be positive. If the shift is to the patient's left, the value will be negative.

Clinical relevance
This measurement is an indicator of global coronal spinal balance.

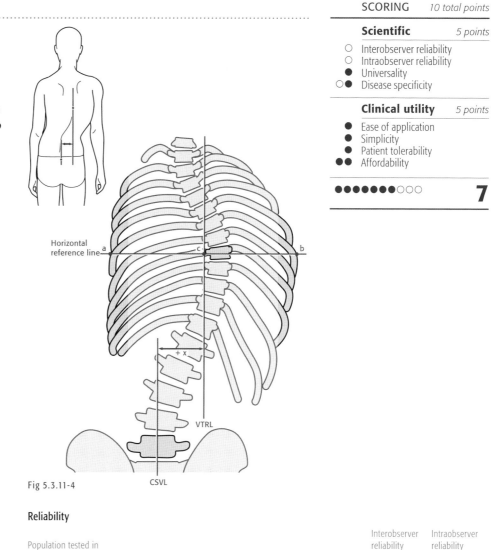

Fig 5.3.11-4

SCORING   *10 total points*

Scientific   *5 points*
○ Interobserver reliability
○ Intraobserver reliability
● Universality
○● Disease specificity

Clinical utility   *5 points*
● Ease of application
● Simplicity
● Patient tolerability
●● Affordability

●●●●●●●○○○   **7**

Reliability

Population tested in	Interobserver reliability	Intraobserver reliability
Not tested		

5.3.12   Axial spinal alignment (rotatory deformity)

1   Angle of trunk inclination

Description
A clinical measurement with the patient flexed forward 90°. The angle created by the horizontal reference line and the line tangential to the trunk rotation is the angle of trunk inclination.

Interpretation
The greater the angle, the greater the rotatory deformity of the spinal column.

Clinical Relevance
This clinical measurement allows the clinician to quantify the severity of rotation within the spinal column deformity.

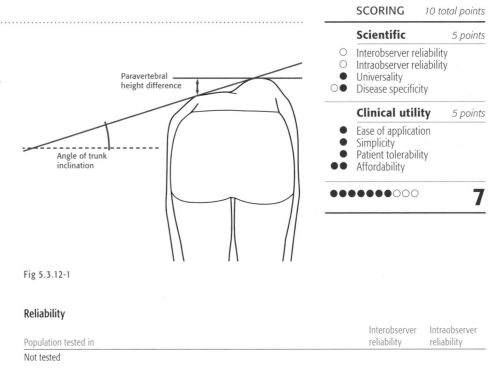

Paravertebral height difference

Angle of trunk inclination

Fig 5.3.12-1

SCORING   *10 total points*

Scientific   *5 points*
○ Interobserver reliability
○ Intraobserver reliability
● Universality
○● Disease specificity

Clinical utility   *5 points*
● Ease of application
● Simplicity
● Patient tolerability
●● Affordability

●●●●●●●○○○   **7**

Reliability

Population tested in	Interobserver reliability	Intraobserver reliability
Not tested		

2   Nash-Moe vertical rotation [1]

Description

A qualitative assessment of the vertebral segment rotation based on the appearance of the pedicles at each individual vertebral segment as viewed on an AP or PA x-ray.

Interpretation

If the appearance of the pedicles is symmetrical, this suggests no rotation of the vertebral body.

The more asymmetrical the appearance of the pedicles on the AP or PA x-ray, the more axially rotated the vertebral body is. In severe rotation, only one pedicle may be visible (Grade III and Grade IV).

Clinical Relevance

This measurement is an indicator of vertebral rotation.

	Concave	Convex
Neutral (0)	No asymmetry	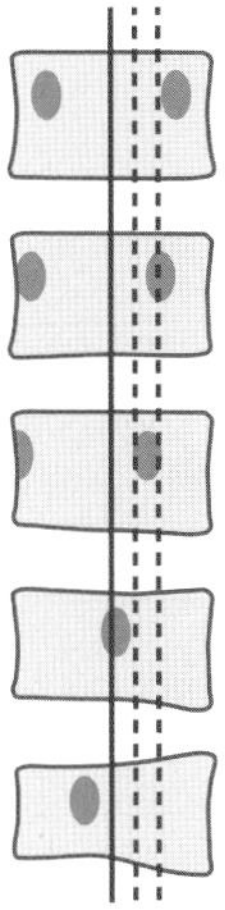 No asymmetry
Grade I	May start disappearing, early distortion	Migrates within first segment, early distortion
Grade II	Gradually disappears	Migrates to second segment
Grade III	Not visible	Migrates to second segment
Grade IV	Not visible	Migrates past midline to concave side of vertebral body

Fig 5.3.12-2

Scientific   *5 points*

○ Interobserver reliability
○ Intraobserver reliability
● Universality
○● Disease specificity

Clinical utility   *5 points*

● Ease of application
● Simplicity
● Patient tolerability
●● Affordability

●●●●●●●○○○   **7**

Reliability

Population tested in	Interobserver reliability	Intraobserver reliability
Spinal x-rays of adolescent idiopathic scoliosis patients (N = 30) were measured twice by 3 fellowship-trained spinal deformity surgeons [2]	-	-

References:
1. Nash CL, Jr., Moe JH (1969) A study of vertebral rotation. *J Bone Joint Surg Am;* 51:223-229.
2. Kuklo TR, Potter BK, Polly DW, Jr., et al (2005) Reliability analysis for manual adolescent idiopathic scoliosis measurements. *Spine;* 30:444-454.

List of assessed measurements

T

U

V

W

Glossary of terms and abbreviations

Terms

Affordability   An estimate of the cost for a measurement compared to the ability of a purchaser to pay for it.

Clinical utility   The extent to which the measurement is useful for a clinician or researcher to make clinical decisions or infer associations. It includes two important characteristics: its simplicity and its ability to direct treatment.

Disease specificity   The accuracy of the measurement in indicating a disease.

Ease of application   The level of difficulty for performing the measurement.

Interobserver reliability   The ability of the measurement to produce the same results with repeat assessment by different observers rating the same severity.

Intraobserver reliability   The ability of the measurement to produce the same results with repeat assessment by the same observer when no important dimension of health has changed.

Methodology   The systematic evaluation of the properties inherent in a measurement. In this context, it refers to the evaluation of a measure's reliability.

Measurement   The process or result of measuring the extent, size, dimensions, capacity, quantity, or volume of the spine or spinal disease (eg, range of motion, vital capacity, muscle strength, Cobb angle). It differs from a severity measure in that measurement does not automatically group disease into categories (see "severity measure").

Outcomes measure   A measure that adequately quantifies the success (or failure) of a treatment intervention.

Patient tolerability   The ability of a patient to tolerate a given measurement.

Population
The group of patients tested in the study and described in terms of the condition (disease or injury), age, and sex.

Reliability   The ability of a measure to produce the same results with repeat assessment by the same observer (intraobserver reliability) or by different observers (interobserver reliability).

Severity measure   A grouping or classification of spinal disease or trauma into categories. These categories may in part be determined by one or more measurements (see "measurement").

Simplicity   The ease of interpretation of the measurement.

Universality   The spectrum of disease for which a measurement can be used.

Abbreviations

ABI	Axis-basion interval	
ADI	Atlantodens interval	
ADP	Air displacement plethysmography	
AFOS	Alkaline phosphatase	
AHI	Apnea-hypopnea index	
ALAT	Alanine aminotransferase	
ALL	Anterior longitudinal ligament	
AOD	Atlantooccipital dislocation	
APCR	Activated protein C resistance	
AS	Ankylosing spondylitis	
ASAT	Aspartate aminotransferase	
ASIA	American spinal injury association	
ATI	Angle of trunk inclination	
AVR	Apical vertebral rotation	
AVT	Apical vertebral translation	
BMC	Bone mineral content	
BMD	Bone mineral density	
BUA	Broadband ultrasound attenuation	
BUN	Blood urea nitrogen	
CBC	Complete blood count	
CBVA	Chin-brow to vertical angle	
CCD	Craniocervical dislocations	
CCP	Cyclic citrullinated peptide	
CSVL	Central sacral vertical line	
CT	Computerized tomography	
CVA	Coronal vertical axis	
DBI	Dens-basion interval	

DEXA or DXA	Dual energy x-ray absorptiometry	
DISH	Diffuse idiopathic skeletal hyperostosis	
dSEP	Dermatomal somatosensory evoked potentials	
DVT	Deep venous thrombosis	
ECHO	Echocardiograms	
EEG	Electroencephalogram	
EGFR	Estimated glomerular filtration rate	
EIA	Enzyme immunoassay	
EMG	Electromyography	
ERV	Expiratory reserve volume	
ESR	Erythrocyte sedimentation rate	
FEV1	Forced expiratory volume in 1 second	
FIM	Functional independence measure	
FRC	Functional residual capacity	
FVC	Forced vital capacity	
GFR	Glomerular filtration rate	
GRASSP	Graded and redefined assessment of strength, sensibility and prehension	
HA	Hip axis	
HCO3	Bicarbonate	
HCT	Hematocrit	
HDL	High-density lipoprotein	
HIV	Human immunodeficiency virus	

IMSOP	International medical society of paraplegia	
INR	International normalized ratio	
IONM	Intraoperative neurophysiological monitoring	
IPA	Interpupillary angle	
JHTF	Jebsen-Taylor hand function test	
LLD	Leg length discrepancy	
MDRD	Modification of diet in renal disease	
MEP	Maximum expiratory pressure	
MIP	Maximum inspiratory pressure	
MMT	Manual motor test	
MRC	Medical research council	
MRI	Magnetic resonance imaging	
NCV	Nerve conduction velocity	
NINDS	National institute of neurologic disorders and stroke	
OPLL	Progression of ossification of the posterior longitudinal ligament	
PaO2	Partial pressure of oxygen in arterial blood	
PCF	Peak cough flows	
PE	Pulmonary embolism	
PI	Pelvic incidence	
PLL	Posterior longitudinal ligament	
PO	Pelvic obliquity	
PSA	Prostate specific antigen	

PSG	Polysomnogram		SVA	Sagittal vertical axis
PT	Pelvic tilt		TAL	Transverse atlantal ligament
PT	Prothrombin time		tcMEP	Transcranial motor evoked potentials
PTH	Parathyroid hormone			
PTT	Partial thromboplastin time		TLC	Total lung capacity
QCT	Quantitative computed tomography		TSH	Thyroid-stimulating hormone
			TUG	Timed up and go test
QIF	Quadriplegia index of function		VEP	Visual evoked potentials
QMA	Quantitative motion analysis		VOS	Velocity of sound
QMT	Quantified muscle test		VTRL	Vertebral trunk reference line
QST	Quantitative sensory test		WB	Western blot
QUS	Quantitative ultrasound		WCC	White cell count
REM	Rapid eye movement		WHO	World health organization
RMI	Rivermead mobility index		WISC-II	Walking index for spinal injury
RV	Residual volume		WMF	Wolf motor function test
SAC	Space available for the cord		6MWT	6-minute walk test
SaO2	Saturation of oxygen in arterial blood		10MWT	10-meter walk test
			10SST	10-second step test
SCI-FAI	Spinal cord injury functional ambulation inventory		30MWT	30-meter walk test
			50FWT	50-foot walk test
SCIM	Spinal cord independence measure			
SEP	Somatosensory evoked potentials			
ShTa	Shoulder tilt angle			
SLE	Systemic lupus erythematosus			
SS	Sacral slope			
STA	Sagittal tilt angle